Evidence Trumps Belief

Nurse Anesthetists and Evidence-Based Decision Making

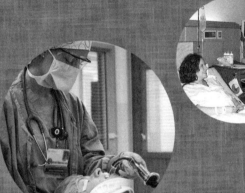

Second Edition

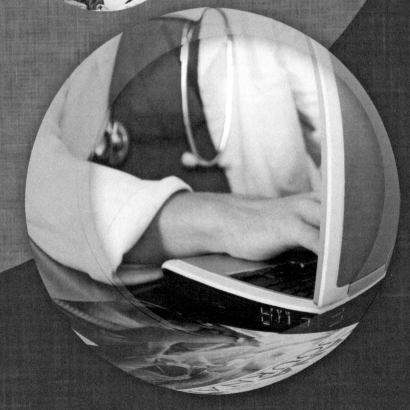

Chuck Biddle

Published by: **American Association of Nurse Anesthetists**

American Association of Nurse Anesthetists
222 South Prospect Avenue
Park Ridge, IL 60068-4001

Printed in the United States of America

Last digit indicates print number: 10 9 8 7 6 5 4 3

Library of Congress Cataloging-in-Publication Data

Biddle, Chuck, 1955- author.
 Evidence trumps belief : nurse anesthetists and evidence-based decision making / by Chuck Biddle. -- [Second edition].
   p. ; cm.
 Includes bibliographical references.
 ISBN 978-0-9829912-0-6 (soft cover)
 I. American Association of Nurse Anesthetists, issuing body. II. Title.
 [DNLM: 1. Nurse Anesthetists. 2. Decision Making. 3. Evidence-Based Nursing. 4. Models, Nursing. 5. Nursing Research. 6. Safety Management. WY 151]
 RD82
 617.9'6--dc23
                                 2013018356

Dedication

This book is dedicated to the patients and students that I have had the privilege of caring for and working with. Both constantly remind me that our daily clinical orbit reveals gaps in knowledge and produces more questions than answers. The responsibility inherent in the practice of nurse anesthesia in closing those gaps and addressing the never-ending stream of questions in the most effective manner possible is at the heart of what we do and is the fuel that impassions me professionally.

Foreword

At some point, the artist must put the paintbrush or mallet and chisel down, and step away, having "finished" the object of his or her attention. Once that happens, as often occurs, a sense of uncertainty, if not downright anxiety sets in at what more could have, or should have, been accomplished. Although not an artist in any sense of the word, I experienced those very sensations at the publication of the first edition, noting omissions and deletions that appeared obvious to me in the rearview mirror.

Embarking on a second edition was fueled, in part, by what I perceive to be pockets of resistance to the tenets of evidence-based decision making (EBDM) that are variably lauded and criticized. The applause comes from those who are wedded to the notion that what we do should be under the strict navigation of objective and sound science. The critics of EBDM are, to my thinking, often blinded to their own biases and seem prone to select out observations, views, and studies that support their preconceived notions of how things should be done.

A study of the critics' arguments leads me to identify 3 major domains of concern that they voiced. (1) Evidence-based decision making is over-reliant on randomized trials. (2) There is insufficient time to accomplish what is required, with associated logistics that are overpowering. (3) The available evidence is often flawed and contradictory.

One aim of this book is to offer objective "evidence" and strategies to counter these arguments. For example: (1) Evidence-based decision making encourages the use of randomized trials and meta-analyses, but in the absence of such evidence the next best level of evidence should be considered. Evidence is hierarchical and contextually sensitive and must be considered as such in rendering any EBDM process. (2) In the 21st century the availability of computers, handheld devices, and customized and efficient electronic search engines defeat concerns of "logistic obstacles" in accessing objective evidence that empowers EBDM. (3) Concerns that the evidence is not perfect are misguided. Given the vicissitudes and complexities inherent in the human condition, the evidence will never be perfect. As one ascends the hierarchy of levels of evidence, the resulting information becomes less prone to bias and serves to shape a clearer picture (always with a need for more refinement!) that approaches the real-world scenarios that clinicians encounter in daily practice.

Challenges abound in understanding and applying EBDM. One of the most formidable involves the problem of evidence failing to penetrate clinical practice. Too often, despite high-quality trials and meta-analyses, best evidence fails to alter real-world practice.

It is my hope that this book will inspire your deep consideration of the principles of EBDM and offer recipes for its successful incorporation into your daily practice. My view is deeply grounded in the notion that whereas EBDM is far from perfect, it is far better than nothing!

Chuck Biddle, CRNA, PhD
Editor in Chief, *AANA Journal*
Professor and Staff Anesthetist
Department of Nurse Anesthesia
Virginia Commonwealth University
Richmond, Virginia

Evidence Trumps Belief: Nurse Anesthetists and Evidence-Based Decision Making

Contents

CHAPTER ONE

The Fabric of Research:
What Gulliver's Voyage Reveals

Certified Registered Nurse Anesthetists (CRNAs) work in one of the most complex and stressful professional domains in existence. The drugs that we use and the interventions that we perform are provided to unique patients, often with challenging comorbidities, who are undergoing psychologically and/or physically painful procedures. We marshal an enormous fund of knowledge and experience to bear on every patient encounter that is unique in its own way. Adding to that mixture are the environmental factors of bewildering technology, multiple team members (eg, surgeons, nurses, and technicians), production pressure, and communication requirements. Although our knowledge comes from a variety of disciplines, including physiology, pharmacology, physics, nursing, medicine, and psychology, research and critical thinking are what make the safe and effective application of our knowledge possible.

In the Jonathan Swift classic, *Gulliver's Travels*, Lemuel Gulliver encounters 4 lands of a peculiar and exotic nature after his shipwrecks. Gulliver, the ship's surgeon and a man of science, arrives at the land of Laputa, a floating island in a vast open space where science functions chaotically and without practical end points. There, fantastic experiments and interventions are under way that will benefit no one (eg, attempts to bottle sunshine for rainy days, making pillows out of marble, and fabricating gunpowder from ice). There are even a few experiments that may cause harm (eg, the search for an ink for inscribing text that when eaten will be retained in one's memory, thus avoiding the need to read or study). The disconnect between the needs of the people and the objectives of science is obvious.

Unlike what Gulliver encountered in Laputa, we depend on research to provide the tools to engage in an efficient and valid approach to making the best practice choices among initially plausible alternatives and to provide a systematic means for assessing their value. Whether selecting an antiemetic, administering an intravenous fluid, deciding on mechanical ventilator settings, or planning postoperative pain control, we rely on research to provide a foundation for clinical decision making, thus avoiding fads and inferior alternatives.

Without question, the dissemination of research findings to anesthesia practitioners is occurring at a higher rate than ever before seen. Not only are the results of research being presented with greater frequency at anesthesia symposia of all kinds, but research is also conspicuous even in publications previously devoted entirely to clinical anesthesia.

The impact of research on the day-to-day activities of CRNAs has become an especially relevant topic. Before the mid-1970s, nearly all nurse anesthetists functioned without much consideration of research, and fewer still engaged in systematic study and subsequent publication of their ideas. In the late 1970s and into the 1980s, the profession experienced a period of punctuated evolution. Major driving forces behind this evolution included movement into a graduate educational framework, more sophisticated appreciation of the scientific underpinnings of our specialty, recognition of the importance of evidence-based decision making (EBDM), national attention to issues of patient outcome and patient safety, and a growing self-awareness of nurse anesthetists not only as providers of excellent clinical care but also as active participant scholars in the domains relevant to anesthesia care. Today, the profession is charged with a new set of challenges (and opportunities) as our university programs produce nurse anesthetists with clinical and research doctoral degrees.

The Process of Research

Certified Registered Nurse Anesthetists primarily function with a practice-oriented perspective; therefore, the recommendations of Brown and colleagues[1] seem especially relevant. These scholars suggest 4 characteristics of research that are vital to the development of a scientific knowledge base for a discipline. First, research should be actively conducted by the members of the discipline. Second, research should be focused on clinical problems encountered by members of the discipline. Third, the approach to these problems must be grounded in a conceptual framework—that is, it must be scientifically based, emphasizing selection, arrangement, and clarification of existing relationships. Fourth, the methods used in studying the problems must be fundamentally sound. To this I would add the need to evaluate the conduct and outcomes of the study in such a way that promotes a continuous search for improving care by revealing new avenues of future research.

How We Come to Know What We Know

As we come to better understand and use EBDM in the care of patients, it is important to recognize how it is that we come to know things, to accept these things as truths, and what factors serve to weaken or strengthen our resolve. *Research* is the application of a systematic approach to the study of a problem or question, but research is not the only way we come to know things. A good deal of our knowledge emerges through *tradition* and *custom*, which are important sources of human knowledge. Americans are raised in a democratic society and, as such, learn that democracy is the best and most advanced form of government. This method is powerful and efficient, but in the absence of evaluating tradition and custom for validity and reliability, it may lead to blind acceptance.

Many of us come to know something to be true because an authoritative person tells us so. This method, *authoritarianism*, suffers because the knowledge passed on remains unchallenged and may be incorrect. Should we not ask the basis for what we are being told? Examples of authorities abound and include parents, teachers, government officials, and the clergy. Clinical and classroom instructors of anesthesia may represent powerful authority figures to students, with the risk of students uncritically embracing all that they are told or shown.

The *trial-and-error method* is a common and quite powerful source of knowledge. In this method, one makes an observation (eg, being in the strong sun too long causes a sunburn) and, on that basis, makes a prediction (eg, the sun is potentially dangerous) and implements subsequent behaviors (eg, avoids the sun or uses protective clothing or sunscreen). However, a risk remains: not only are certain events perceived differently by different people, but also one person's experience may be too narrow to serve as the basis for the development of a reasonable and unbiased understanding of a given phenomenon. Although this mechanism is a practical way of knowing, it is highly fallible and represents a coarse, inefficient, and potentially dangerous way to gain knowledge.

Logical reasoning represents another way of knowing. The reasoning method has 2 components: inductive reasoning and deductive reasoning. *Inductive reasoning* results in generalizations that are derived from specific observations. Consider the following line of reasoning using Rambo, Sylvester Stallone's character in several action movies, as an example. We observe that Rambo is mortal; we observe that a number of other people are mortal as well; on this basis, we conclude that all people are mortal. *Deductive reasoning* is the development of specific predictions from generalities. In this case, we see the following line of reasoning: we know that all men are mortal; we know that Rambo is a man; therefore, we conclude that Rambo is mortal. Both methods are useful, but the former offers no mechanism for evaluation or self-correction, and the latter is not, in itself, a source of new information.

Perhaps the most advanced way of knowing is reflected in the *scientific method*. Although it too is fallible, the scientific method's reliability and validity are generally recognized as exceeding those of other methods. It provides for self-evaluation with a system of checks and balances that minimizes bias, provides control, and limits faulty reasoning. In essence, it is a systematic approach to solving problems and enhancing our understanding of phenomena. It has, at its foundation, the gathering and interpretation of information without prejudice.

Research as a Professional Tool to Refine and Seek Knowledge

Research is, by definition, a dynamic phenomenon. Whether it is directed purely at the acquisition of knowledge for knowledge's sake (basic research) or at the specific solution of problems (applied research), it is a process that is systematic and discovery oriented.

Although research can assume many forms, it must be valid, internally and externally. *Internal validity* is the researcher's control of and the power of the relationship among variables in the study and the study's measured outcome. It is a necessary but not sufficient condition for ensuring external validity. *External validity* is an application issue, that is, to whom the results of the study can be applied. *Reliability* refers to the extent that data collection, analysis, and interpretation are consistent and helps to define one's confidence that the research can be replicated and similar conclusions reached. When research works well, it represents a systematic approach that includes the identification of the problem or problems, the gathering and critical review of relevant information, the collection of data in a highly defined and orchestrated manner, the analysis of the data appropriate to the problem or problems faced, and the development of conclusions within the framework of the study.

Science is not a routine, cut-and-dried process. Rather, scientific knowledge emerges from an enterprise that is intensely human, and, as a consequence, it is subject to the full spectrum of human strengths and limitations; paramount among the limitations is bias.

Critical Stages in the Research Process

Research must be logical, progress in an orderly manner, and, ultimately, be grounded within the framework of the scientific method. If research is a way of searching for truths, revealing solutions to problems, and generating principles that result in theories, we must come to understand the process of research. Having a good appreciation of this process will better equip us as we engage in EBDM.

The research process can be described in many ways. For purposes of simplicity, this process comprises 8 mutually exclusive, but interdependent, essential stages:

1. Identification of the problem
2. Review of the relevant knowledge and literature
3. Formulation of the hypothesis or research question
4. Development of an approach for testing the hypothesis
5. Execution of the research plan
6. Analysis and interpretation of the data
7. Dissemination of the findings to interested colleagues
8. Evaluation of the research report

As will be evident later, these critical steps in the research process have considerable overlap and similarity to the steps associated with evidence-based practice. Just as we encounter a wide range of patient challenges, we constantly encounter problems and situations that are in need of interrogation in a systematic manner. For example, in the lounge during a conversation with colleagues or at a clinical anesthesia conference, one hears remarks such as the following:

- "A 50-mg dose of thiopental given just before propofol alleviates virtually any pain on injection."
- "Do you think there is less nausea and vomiting in healthy outpatients who are deliberately overhydrated?"

- "I find that the use of the waveform generated by my pulse oximeter yields valuable information regarding depth of anesthesia."
- "I believe that use of the inspiratory pause mechanism available on the Ohmeda 7810 ventilator significantly improves arterial oxygen tension in patients with chronic obstructive pulmonary disease."
- "I am convinced that [the anesthesia provider's] sleepiness is a major cause of anesthesia accidents."
- "Lactated Ringer's solution can be used to dilute packed red blood cells if only 100 mL is added to each unit of cells."
- "Ultrasound-guided regional anesthesia is associated with fewer adverse effects than landmark or nerve stimulator approaches."
- "It is OK to write with a felt pen on a plastic bag of intravenous fluid."

A problem that lends itself to research often materializes from personal observations and in the sharing of ideas and experiences among people who are familiar with the phenomenon in question. Likewise, such questions urge consideration on the individual patient level, thus inviting application of the principles of evidence-based practice.

The wording of the problem statement sets the stage for the type of study design and analysis that are used. A study reported in 2007 in the journal *Anesthesiology* by Myles et al[2] assessed the length of hospital stay (a common outcome closely associated with complications) in patients who received or did not receive nitrous oxide. Although no difference was found in the stated objective, the authors then used secondary measures (eg, death and myocardial infarction) to build a case against the use of nitrous oxide, measures that the study was not well suited to measure. The study received severe criticism for this as well as the use of these secondary measures and for other methodologic flaws.

Each step in the research process subsequently influences later steps. A mistake made early on inevitably creates difficulties at a later stage in the process.

Research Methods

The research method is the way the truth of a phenomenon is coaxed from the world in which it resides, free of the biases of the human condition. Just as we have a vast array of drugs and approaches that we choose from to individualize anesthetic care, investigators have at their disposal a variety of research methods so that they are not inflexibly wedded to any particular approach. Researchers do not follow a single scientific method but, rather, have at their disposal an array of methods that are amenable to their field of study.

Some of the methods available are highly recognizable, permanent components of a researcher's armamentarium, whereas others have evolved with respect to time and in response to the specific needs of a particular problem or discipline. The research method can be influenced by the way a researcher views a problem. For example, a researcher can test a hypothesis, search for a correlation, ask "why" or "how" questions, or probe a phenomenon on the basis of "what would happen if" suppositions. The nature of the question or questions asked and the research design used have considerable influence on a practitioner's decision to use findings in an evidence-based approach.

The research method can be characterized by its temporal relationship to the problem. A *retrospective study* is the process of surveying the past: the phenomenon in which we are interested has already occurred, and we are simply looking to see what occurred. This type of design lends itself well to establishing associations between variables for interventions and outcomes, but it is not appropriate for defining cause-and-effect relationships. In contrast, a *prospective study* sets out to see what will happen following an intervention; the collection of data proceeds forward in time and, with proper controls (discussed later in this section), allows for cause-and-effect relationships to be identified.

It is important to understand several terms that are fundamental to the research process. The *dependent variable* is the object of the study or that variable being measured. The *independent variable* is the variable that is primarily under study (and is often directly manipulated) and is presumed to cause or influence the dependent variable. Another way of looking at this relationship is that variables that are consequences of or are dependent on antecedent variables are considered dependent variables.

Another set of variables is known as *control variables* and as *background* or *attribute variables*. Control variables are not actively manipulated by the researcher, but because they might influence relationships under study, they must be controlled, held constant, or randomized so that their effects are neutralized, canceled out, or at least considered by the researcher. Consider a study that proposes to examine the efficacy and safety of interscalene regional anesthesia using ultrasound or electrical nerve stimulation to target the location for local anesthetic injection. The independent variable would be the approach (ultrasound vs electrical nerve stimulation), and the dependent variable would be an outcome (eg, quality of the block, time to complete block, or adverse events) resulting from the intervention. A number of control variables (eg, who administered the block, the dose and type of local anesthetic, and patient factors) would need to be accounted for, because they might, if not controlled in some manner, influence the outcome measures.

Blinding (or *masking*) is the process of controlling for obvious and occult bias arising from subjects' or researchers' reactions to what is going on. In a *single-blind* design, patients are unaware which treatment or manipulation is being given to them. In a *double-blind* design, neither research observers or recorders nor patients are aware of the treatment or manipulation being given. In a *triple-blind* design, patients, observers, and people involved in the final data analysis are not aware of the actual treatment or manipulation being applied. Whereas *randomization* attempts to equalize the groups at the start of the study, blinding further equalizes the groups by controlling for psychological biases that might arise apart from any effect of the treatment. Many factors influence the decision whether to use a single-blind, double-blind, or triple-blind design. The degree of study rigor and consideration given to issues involving bias are major factors to consider for researchers, as well as anesthesia providers—the ultimate consumers of the research report that emerges.

Recently, a newer term is gaining more widespread use in the biomedical literature—the *double-dummy* design, also referred to as the *double-placebo* design. This approach is generally used in drug intervention studies in which participants receive the assigned active drug and the placebo matched to the comparison drug. Such trials involve 2 active drugs and 2 matching placebos. For example, in comparing 2 drugs, one in a green capsule and the other in an orange capsule, the investigator would acquire green placebo capsules and orange placebo capsules. This approach is believed to improve the double-blinding process.

In many situations, disguising the treatment intervention may prove challenging or even impossible. For example, in a study involving a comparison of general anesthesia with a regional anesthetic approach to hip joint arthroplasty, shielding the patient or the outcome assessor from the intervention is likely impossible.

Classifying Research on the Basis of Methodology

There are many classification schemes for research design. Ultimately, the research design is one that is dependent on and inextricably wedded to the study's purpose, its scope, and the nature of the problem at hand (**Table 1.1**). The following discussion provides a brief overview of major research design classifications and is meant to assist readers in identifying the strengths and weaknesses of the individual approaches. Much weight is applied to the type of research method used when assessing its rigor and its relevance to EBDM.

Research designs can be classified into 2 broad domains: experimental and observational. *Observational studies* do not involve an investigator-controlled manipulation or intervention, but rather simply track the subjects for a defined period, recording events defined by the researcher's objectives. The independent variable (eg, a clinical intervention such as a patient who received or did not receive a blood transfusion for aortic valve surgery as part of routine care) is simply a matter of record, and a dependent variable (eg, an outcome such as rate of wound infection or fever) is recorded. Such a study can progress forward in time (prospective) or, in the case of a look-back (retrospective) study, examine an institutional database. Another type of observational study is the cross-sectional study, in which well-defined measures are recorded at predetermined time points.

Case reports are commonly seen in the anesthesia literature and provide an opportunity to vicariously experience the care provided to a patient but are subject to substantial bias. We learn about the perioperative events and characteristics of an individual patient (or of a series of similar patients in a "case series") and of the successes or failures associated with a described management regimen. At best, this type of design is used to generate a hypothesis because the design does not allow for the controls necessary for hypothesis testing.

The *case-control study* is a type of observational study (**Figure 1.1**). An outcome that has occurred is identified (eg, blindness following anesthesia), and the researcher looks back to identify factors that seem to be associated with the outcome. A key component

Table 1.1. Brief Synopsis of Major Study Designs

Study design	Advantages	Disadvantages
Survey	• Generally inexpensive and simple • Low risk of ethical problems	• Establishment of association at best; no demonstration of cause and effect • Susceptible to recall bias • Possible unequal distribution of confounders between or among groups • Possible unequal group sizes
Case-control study	• Generally quick and inexpensive • Feasible method for studying very rare disorders or disorders with long lag between exposure and outcome • Fewer subjects needed than cross-sectional studies	• Reliance on recall or records to determine exposure status • Confounders difficult to identify and control • Possible difficulty in selection of control groups • Large risk of bias: recall, selection
Cohort study	• Ethically safe • Matched subjects • Can establish timing and directionality of events • Can standardize eligibility criteria and outcome assessments • Administratively easier and less expensive than randomized controlled trials	• Possible difficulty identifying control subjects • Exposure possibly linked to a hidden confounder • Difficulty in blinding • Lack of randomization • For rare disease, large sample or long follow-up necessary
Randomized controlled trial	• Unbiased distribution of confounders • Blinding more likely • Statistical analysis facilitated by randomization	• Expensive in terms of time and money • Volunteer bias—not all patients willing to be "randomized" • Ethically problematic at times

Table continues on page 9.

Table 1.1. Brief Synopsis of Major Study Designs

Study design	Advantages	Disadvantages
Observational study	• No random assignment • Generally inexpensive	• Loss of control over the intervention • Loss of control over potential (known and unknown) confounders
Retrospective design	• Cheaper and generally easier to perform than prospective studies • Highly useful for discerning the nature of phenomena, especially in describing associations between or among variables • Improved techniques and statistical methods have made these methods more defensible • Data often housed in existing manual or electronic databases, making access convenient	• Independent variable has already occurred • Loss of control over variables • Cannot ascertain cause-and-effect relationships • Determining which variable is dependent and which is independent not consistently possible when a relationship is revealed
Crossover design	• Smaller sample needed because subjects serve as own controls and error variance is reduced • All subjects receive treatment (at least some of the time) • Statistical tests assuming randomization can be used • Blinding can be maintained	• All subjects receive placebo or alternative treatment at some point • Lengthy or unknown washout period (recovery from a given intervention) • Not usable for treatments with permanent effects

of the design is the identification of a similar group of patients who did not experience the negative outcome. This component is called matching, usually with respect to the patients' gender, age, surgical procedure, and other factors. By controlling for these factors, the baseline characteristics of the comparison populations are balanced or equalized, allowing for improved opportunity to identify factors that may be associated with

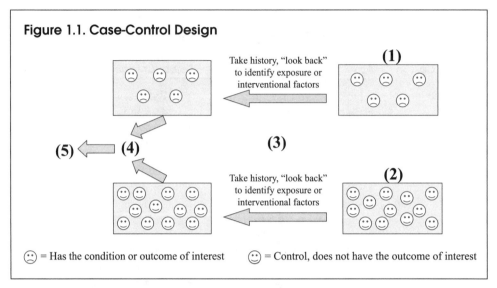

Figure 1.1. Case-Control Design

⊙⊙ = Has the condition or outcome of interest   ⊙⊙ = Control, does not have the outcome of interest

Begin with a group of patients who have the outcome or condition (1). Compare a larger, matched group who do not have the outcome or condition (2). Search for differences between the groups to look at factors that may be associated with the outcome (3). Draw conclusions (4). Set the stage for prospective study (5).

the negative outcome. Traditionally, this type of study is considered sufficiently powered if the ratio of cases (people who experienced the bad outcome) to controls (people who did not experience the bad outcome) is 1:2 or greater (1:3 or 1:4 is optimal). Case-control studies are useful for identifying associations between a variable (or variables) and an outcome but are not powerful enough to allow for cause and effect to be determined.

Loss of control over factors that influence the outcome predominates in observational studies. A researcher has no control over the treatment assigned to a patient, there is no control over the numerous variables likely to affect the outcome of interest, and many forms of bias sum to produce results that, at best, allow associations to emerge between described variables. One tool used to improve on the validity of conclusions reached from observational studies is the use of *propensity score analysis,* discussed in Chapter 3.

Experimental research designs are prospective and involve some type of intervention. The goal is to describe and assess an approach for its safety or efficacy or to determine if one approach offers benefit over existing interventions. A *cohort study* is a prospective study that follows up a group or groups of patients over time who have a certain condition and/or receive a particular treatment; the data for the subjects then are compared with those for another group who lack the condition or are not receiving the treatment under investigation. Cohort studies work well for experiments that might otherwise be unethical or dangerous. For example, such a study might identify, in advance, 2 groups of patients undergoing laparoscopic gallbladder surgery: a group of people who are morbidly obese and a comparison group of people who are not. Following them forward in time and assessing certain outcomes such as difficulty in intubation, drug requirements, duration of surgery, positioning-related injury, ventilatory requirements, and other out-comes would allow some general conclusions to be reached regarding considerations in caring for patients undergoing a similar procedure, yet with markedly different body habitus.

The gold standard of clinical, experimental research is the randomized controlled clinical trial. Clinical trials, by definition, involve the use of humans as subjects and require a specific set of criteria (**Figure 1.2**). Because there are powerful controls established and the element of bias is reduced, we are better able to reveal the true effect of an intervention on selected measured outcomes. As will be evident, randomized trials are heavily relied on in developing a best evidence approach to decision making for patient care.

Quasi-experimental research differs from experimental research in that it is missing one or more of the key elements required for the experimental design. For example, at an institution, outpatients may routinely receive ondansetron from practitioner *X,* whereas they routinely do not receive ondansetron from practitioner *Y.* A prospective trial in which both practitioners use a standard anesthetic technique could be initiated. For example, sevoflurane in 50% nitrous oxide, fentanyl, and rocuronium could be administered as the general anesthetic regimen, allowing practitioners *X* and *Y* to use or not use ondansetron as they usually would. Outcome, measured by the incidence of nausea and vomiting in the first 6 postoperative hours, is quantified, and the groups are compared. Although randomization is not achieved, a study that may not have been possible because of the inflexibility of the clinicians involved is successfully accomplished. Quasi-experiments, by yielding to one or more of the rigid criteria of the experimental design, offer an attractive alternative in certain circumstances. However, researchers

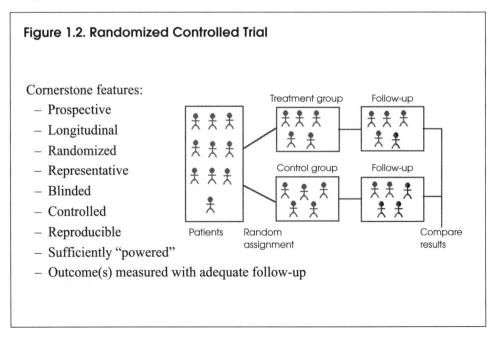

Figure 1.2. Randomized Controlled Trial

Cornerstone features:
- Prospective
- Longitudinal
- Randomized
- Representative
- Blinded
- Controlled
- Reproducible
- Sufficiently "powered"
- Outcome(s) measured with adequate follow-up

Treatment group   Follow-up

Control group   Follow-up

Patients   Random assignment   Compare results

must acknowledge and account for any influence that the quasi-experimental design might have had on what was observed.

Threats to Internal Validity

The sine qua non of research is establishing a relationship of an independent variable (such as a factor or an intervention) to a dependent variable (an outcome of some sort). Anything that threatens that relationship serves to threaten the worth of the entire study. **Table 1.2** summarizes the major categories of threats to the validity of a study's design and notes the associated attributes of the threats.

Qualitative Research: An Alternative Paradigm

Up to this point, the traditional approach to a problem has been characterized by deductive reasoning, objectivity, manipulation, and control. An alternative approach involves a group of methods characterized by inductive reasoning, subjectivity, exploration, and process orientation. These methods fall under the rubric of *qualitative research* techniques.

Table 1.2. Threats to Internal Validity of a Study Design

Internal validity: Are the study design and its methods sensitive enough to detect, measure, and control for the true relationship between the identified independent variable or variables and the identified dependent variable or variables?

History	Events external to the intervention that may affect the outcome
Maturation	Normal physiological and psychological changes that occur during the study that may affect the outcome
Testing	A pretreatment or pretest may alter subsequent measures, regardless of the intervention
Instrumentation	Inconsistencies with the testing or measurement instrument, including the individuals using it
Statistical regression	Natural tendency for people who score or who are measured at the extremes (high or low) to move closer to the mean when subsequently retested
Mortality	Death of subjects (for any reason) during the study
Selection	Differences (known and unknown) in the subjects that exist before the start of the study
Interactivity of selection with aforementioned factors	Certain characteristics of the subjects in the study are confused with a treatment (intervention) effect; may be due to differential effects in subject selection factors

Qualitative techniques include philosophic inquiry, histography, phenomenology, grounded theory, and ethnography. Generally speaking, qualitative research refers to systematic modes of inquiry directed principally at observing, describing, analyzing, interpreting, and understanding the patterns, themes, qualities, and meanings of specific contextual phenomena. Qualitative research seeks to gain insight by discovering the meanings associated with a given phenomenon and exploring the depth, richness, and complexity inherent in it.

For example, exploring how male and female CRNAs differ in the manner in which they deal with parental and child separation discomfort when a child is readied for induction of anesthesia might best be achieved through the use of a qualitative design. The actual experiences might be observed or videotaped. Those involved—anesthetists, parents, and children—might be interviewed immediately and at some time thereafter, using open-ended questions that allow themes or patterns of behaviors to emerge. Another example is a study of the impact of a natural disaster (eg, Hurricane Katrina or Ike) on the provision of anesthesia care in the Gulf of Mexico area during and in the immediate aftermath. Those involved—anesthetists and anesthesiologists—might be interviewed to assess their individual and collective "lived experiences" of this time. Both studies would be artificially constrained and disjointed if conducted in any setting other than the original or if too many controls were brought to bear on the experiment.

The qualitative paradigm seems especially apropos when a researcher does not want to artificially distance a study from its contextual richness or when there is not enough information available on a particular subject for the adequate development of sound and testable hypotheses. The treatise on qualitative approaches by Marshall and Rossman[3] is recommended to interested readers.

In general, qualitative research approaches tend to be best suited to address a research question or function as a hypothesis-generating process. An example of this latter function, and one of the first qualitative studies published in the anesthesia literature, was the sentinel study by Caplan et al[4] examining unexpected cardiac arrest during spinal anesthesia. This qualitative study, using a closed-claims database, revealed a host of themes and patterns of clinical care that were associated with the onset of cardiac arrest with catastrophic outcome. Although not hypothesis-testing in design or intent, the study paved the way for subsequent hypothesis-testing research and served as a major player in establishing an evidence-based approach, during regional anesthesia, to improving patient safety.

Sampling

Under most circumstances, studying everyone who might be affected by a particular study is impractical, if not impossible. For example, if we want to know how effective intravenous nitroglycerin is in minimizing the rise in blood pressure associated with laryngoscopy in hypertensive patients, we cannot realistically study all hypertensive patients who undergo laryngoscopy. Rather, we would hope to find a smaller group of subjects who are representative of the relevant population at large. By accessing certain information in the sample, we can credibly make inferences or generalizations about the population at large.

Similarly, if we want to know how often anesthesia machines in community hospitals receive preventive maintenance, we cannot visit all community hospitals nationwide. Rather, we might randomly select a number of hospitals in a number of different states, visit those locations, and inspect the maintenance records. By studying a truly representative sample, we can make some reasonable and safe generalizations about the phenomenon of preventive maintenance at large.

Sampling affects many issues related to the process of EBDM, including such questions as the following:

- Are the subjects in the study representative of the patients I encounter?
- Are there enough subjects in the study groups to provide sufficient statistical power for the investigation?
- Is there diversity in attributes within the sample, and, if so, are the attributes evenly distributed between or among the study's treatment arms?

In reality, we rarely find a truly random sample from the population at large in a study. More likely, we encounter a *convenience sample,* one chosen largely on the basis of accessibility, expediency, and cost; usually this means that it involves subjects or patients who are available and approachable.

For example, in a study designed to quantify the rate of arterial desaturation in pediatric patients undergoing tonsillectomy who are transported to the postanesthesia care unit with and without supplemental oxygen, the researcher is limited to the patients who are undergoing surgery at the institution or institutions available. It would be impossible to obtain a sample from the population of children at large and subject them to anesthesia and surgery! Rather, a convenience sample consisting of pediatric patients who are having the procedure at the involved institution is used. However, researchers would *randomly assign* study participants to 1 of 2 treatment groups—a group receiving supplemental oxygen or a group not receiving supplemental oxygen—to strengthen the study design.

Obtaining a true random sample, especially in clinical research, is often a complicated if not dauntingly impossible process. More realistic is ensuring random assignment to the study's treatment arms. Most important is the realization that the concept of randomness is essential to minimizing human biases associated with selection and assignment when conducting and interpreting clinical research. Randomization in clinical trials is an essential ingredient in evaluating any study for its validity and is an important criterion for weighing the worth of the study findings in any evidence-based approach to care.

Instrumentation and Measurement

Two important concepts essential to measurement are validity and reliability. Instrument *validity* is the degree to which an instrument, such as a blood pressure cuff or a personality inventory, measures what one believes it is measuring. Instrument *reliability* refers to the degree of consistency with which an instrument measures whatever it is measuring (ie, whether the same result is obtained in repeated trials).

Validity and reliability are often easily established for measures of certain physiologic phenomena but may be troublesome in behavioral or psychological evaluations. Imagine trying to determine reliability and validity for a thermometer. Contrast this with trying to establish validity and reliability for a psychological tool that professes to measure a CRNA's attitude as it relates to providing anesthesia care for a woman undergoing an abortion; obviously, the latter is a much more difficult undertaking. Although a measure must be reliable to be valid, it can be reliable without being valid. For example, a skin temperature probe might reliably (consistently) measure temperature, even in a variety of extreme settings, although it might not be viewed as a valid indicator of core temperature. Reliability and validity are discussed in degrees rather than in all-or-none terms.

When evaluating the findings of a study, it is critical to consider whether the reliability and validity of its outcome measures were established. For example, if an instrument measures evoked responses in the esophagus as a monitor of depth of anesthesia, it must be determined whether the reliability and validity of the instrument have been established under the conditions of the anesthetic protocol being used in the proposed study. Studies of pain management, postoperative nausea and vomiting, difficulty of airway management, and other clinically important domains must strive to demonstrate to readers that the outcome measure is assessed in a stringent manner that is associated with a high degree of validity and reliability. If a researcher fails to establish reliability and validity, the results must be viewed as suspect at best.

Occasionally, a researcher may encounter no reasonable measures to use for a study. For example, instruments for measuring such phenomena as arterial oxygen tension, end-tidal anesthetic concentration, and opioid metabolic by-products are well established. A researcher may need to develop a totally new instrument to determine clinicians' perceptions regarding the propriety of a drug company's high-pressure promotional campaigns for its newly released pharmaceutical product. In developing such a tool, it is helpful to have an expert in the discipline review the instrument, in this case likely a survey tool of some kind, and provide feedback to ensure that the instrument is appropriate. Subsequent to this review, a small pilot study might be conducted to test the tool in a setting that mimics the planned full study to further assess its usefulness and worth.

In designing a study, a researcher must decide how best to measure a phenomenon such as anxiety level, blood pressure, attitude toward healthcare, or rate of complications. In evaluating a study for inclusion in an evidence-based decision-making process, we must decide if the investigator demonstrated that the outcome measures were valid and reliable.

Human Subjects Committee and Institutional Review Board

Federal regulations and individual institutions (eg, universities and medical centers) require that research involving humans be reviewed and approved by an institutional review board (IRB), a human subjects committee (HSC), or some other formal committee to ensure that the proposed research is ethical and does not expose the research stakeholders to unnecessary risk or harm. The concept of *stakeholder* is defined as who (or what) in the conduct of the research might be knowingly or unknowingly placed at risk. Generally, the stakeholders in any planned study include the subjects of the research, the researchers themselves, and the institutions associated with the research.

Most institutions formalize the definitions of research and human subjects, examples of which might include the following:

Research implies a systematic investigation, including some form of development, testing, and evaluation, intended to advance or contribute to generalizable knowledge. A *human subject* is a living (or deceased) person about whom an investigator conducting research obtains data through intervention or interaction with the person or from identifiable private information such as a medical record or database. Some examples of activities that fall under the umbrella of human subjects research include but are not limited to the following:

- Physical interventions applied to the subject
- Adjusting or changing the subject's environment
- Interviews, surveys, and other forms of acquiring information from a subject
- Gathering information about people that was originally obtained for purposes other than a specific research study
- Obtaining body samples such as cells, blood, or tissue
- Access to medical records and data through some type of information system

Once an investigator or team of investigators proposes to perform research as defined, the research protocol must be submitted to the institution's IRB or HSC for full review, and the researchers must await formal approval before any research with human subjects or records of human subjects can proceed. If the research involves animals, there is often a separate committee or a subcommittee of the institution's primary IRB or HSC.

Virtually all journals (including the *AANA Journal*) have stringent requirements for formal documentation of IRB or HSC approval before manuscripts involving research using human subjects undergo review. Readers should familiarize themselves with their own institution's policies because requirements often vary somewhat from one setting to another.

Conclusion

This chapter briefly reviewed some of the major elements of the research process. Information gleaned from basic science and clinical research is optimally applied to the care of patients when done in an evidence-based manner. Fundamental to being an evidence-based nurse anesthetist is having a foundational understanding of what research is, how it should be conducted, and the issues that are involved in its interpretation and translation into meaningful practice applications. As noted at the start of this chapter, although Gulliver found a bewildering and disheartening disconnect between research and practice during his miraculous voyage, evidence-based practice is, as we shall see, a method whose intent is to build connectivity between well-conducted research and the ultimate consumers—patients.

References

1. Brown J, Tanner CA, Padrick KP. Nursing's search for scientific knowledge. *Nurs Res.* 1984;33(1):26-32.

2. Myles PS, Leslie K, Chan MT, et al; for ENIGMA Trial Group. Avoidance of nitrous oxide for patients undergoing major surgery: a randomized controlled trial. *Anesthesiology.* 2007;107(2):221-231.

3. Marshall C, Rossman G. *Designing Qualitative Research.* 4th ed. London, England: Sage Publications; 2006.

4. Caplan RA, Ward RJ, Posner K, Cheney FW. Unexpected cardiac arrest during spinal anesthesia: a closed claims analysis of predisposing factors. *Anesthesiology.* 1988;68(1):5-11.

CHAPTER TWO

So You Want to Be an Evidence-Based Anesthetist?

Although based on several essential tenets, evidence-based practice and evidence-based decision making (EBDM) can assume a variety of forms, and no one approach is necessarily applicable or ideal to all situations. The first crucial step in any evidence-based undertaking is to ask yourself 2 questions: "Do I want to be an evidence-based anesthetist?" and "Am I willing to challenge my own anesthesia care-related decisions in a sincere manner?" Evidence-based practice and decision making are active, not passive, processes requiring commitment and adherence to certain principles that result in uniquely focused decision making about patient care in the context of specific clinical circumstances. Fundamentally, the approach hinges on the desire of individual anesthetists to make judgments based on scientifically valid information in conjunction with their own experience and expertise.

Consider this. In 2003, a sentinel publication revealed that only about half of American citizens receive treatment consistent with state-of-the-art knowledge.[1] The Institute of Medicine's landmark report of the state of US healthcare observed a virtual chasm between services that are delivered and services that are available.[2] Consider also that more than 90 million Americans have at least 1 chronic medical condition, and many have 2 or more. Chronic conditions account for about 75% of all healthcare expenditures.[3]

Think of some of the variations in practice among your colleagues and mentors that you observe relative to the following:

- Prophylaxis for nausea and vomiting
- Blunting of the sympathetic response to laryngoscopy
- The use of regional anesthesia in patients taking substances that impair coagulation
- The way in which arms are padded (or not) and positioned during surgery
- The use (or not) of convective body warmers and fluid warmers
- The transfusion of whole blood and its components
- The way that the care of children with an upper respiratory tract infection is managed
- The manner in which the care of a patient with obstructive sleep apnea is managed
- Allowing (or not) parents to attend pediatric anesthetic inductions
- The type and amount of intravenous fluid administered

- The choice of the fraction of inspired oxygen during routine general anesthesia
- The use of nitrous oxide
- The use of muscle relaxants
- Postoperative pain therapy
- The use (or not) of sighs during routine mechanical ventilation
- The use (or not) of mechanical ventilation with a laryngeal mask airway
- The use (or not) of preemptive analgesia
- The use (or not) of supplemental oxygen postoperatively
- The use of antifibrinolytics to reduce blood loss in cardiothoracic surgery
- Cuffed vs uncuffed endotracheal tubes in infants and small children

Many factors influence variability in clinical practice. Many decisions seem to be grounded more in entrenched belief than firmly rooted in scientifically conducted research. We do something a certain way because that is how we learned in school. We believe that our approach is favorable to that of others. We do something because we have always done it that way. We heard about a success story from another colleague and want to try it. We read an article advocating a certain approach and want to try it. We had a recent failure with an approach and abandoned or changed the approach on the spot. Then, of course, there is variability because some embrace an intervention on the basis of compelling evidence that has application in the unique and context-sensitive situation of a particular patient.

So, you have decided that you want your nurse anesthesia practice to be evidence based. You want to marshal the very best, sound decision making for your patient care. Once you have decided that EBDM is the way to go, you must be prepared to do the following:

1. Ask the right questions.
2. Seek information that critically addresses each question.
3. Evaluate the information retrieved.
4. Implement the plan with the patient or patient population under consideration.
5. Evaluate the intervention.

Asking the Right Questions

It is no small feat, yet an essential component of evidence-based practice, to compose an appropriate question for research and clinical practice. The vital attributes of a well-written evidence-based practice question include the following:

1. The patient (or group) under consideration
2. The intervention to be applied (and a comparison intervention if one is being considered)
3. The outcome to be measured
4. A focus on a clinically relevant issue

The question drives the subsequent steps in any evidence-based practice approach and, in no small part, guides the fate of the inquiry. A couple of sample questions follow:

In a child with cerebral palsy, is the use of succinylcholine associated with an increase in the serum potassium level?

In an adult with obstructive sleep apnea undergoing tonsillectomy and uvulectomy, is the intraoperative use of ketorolac plus fentanyl associated with greater blood loss compared with the use of only fentanyl?

The major goals in developing the question include carefully describing the patient or patient group receiving care; defining the primary intervention planned for use, including a comparison intervention if appropriate; and specifying the major outcome effect under consideration. Careful attention to these goals will greatly assist in keeping the question focused and clinically relevant.

The PICO Approach

A common model used in developing an appropriate clinical question is the PICO approach. PICO is a mnemonic that describes key components to good question construction: *p*atient, *i*ntervention (or cause), *c*omparison (if appropriate), and *o*utcome. Because clinical circumstances and their associated questions vary considerably, not all questions will have a "comparison" group, although many will. **Table 2.1** shows 3 examples of PICO-derived questions.

Table 2.1. PICO Question Examples

Patient	Intervention	Comparison	Outcome
61-year-old man, infarction	Streptokinase	Plasminogen activator	Death
31-year-old woman, laparoscopy	Ondansetron, 4 mg	Droperidol, 1.25 mg	Nausea
17-year-old boy, arthroscopy	Spinal anesthesia		Time in the postanesthesia care unit

By using the PICO approach, a clinically focused, relevant question emerges from each of the scenarios. For example, with respect to the second patient mentioned in Table 2.1, a comparison scenario, the following question might emerge:

In young women undergoing diagnostic laparoscopy and anesthesia with sevoflurane, atracurium, and fentanyl, for evaluation of nonspecific pelvic pain, is there a difference in the rate of postoperative nausea when ondansetron, 4 mg, or droperidol, 1.25 mg, is given 30 minutes before emergence?

With respect to the third patient, a noncomparison question, the following question might emerge:

In adolescents undergoing knee arthroscopy under spinal anesthesia with lidocaine, 75 mg, and sufentanil, 10 µg, what is the anticipated length of stay in the postanesthesia care unit (PACU)?

For readers interested in a free electronic tool to assist in developing PICO-based queries, PICOmaker is a Palm OS–based application that lets users create and store queries in the PICO format for later reference. The tool is designed to assist students and clinicians with processes related to evidence-based practice and can be accessed at http://www.usc.edu/hsc/ebnet/ebframe/PICO.htm.

Seeking Information That Critically Addresses the Question

Once the question is established, it is time to search for relevant and sound information that will facilitate arriving at its answer. I think of this phase of the process as similar to a desire to get into shape. This can mean many things to different people, with the approach varying considerably (from every-other-day walks to hiring a full-time personal fitness trainer) for the intended outcome. In our case, we have a goal of achieving the best evidence, so the bar is set pretty high for us (and our patients).

Seeking the evidence that addresses the question can take many forms: reading the relevant pages in a textbook, discussing the question with a respected colleague, reading an article or two that comes to mind, quickly scanning an electronic database, or immersion in a quest to find every study and review article published that bears on the question. With each of these approaches, there are problems and issues. The ultimate approach taken is as much a matter of commitment to seeking the best evidence as it is to the logistics of time and resources that can be mustered. For EBDM to have a secure and practical place in a busy clinician's professional life, I recommend a pragmatic compromise so that it does not become an ineffective, superficial process or one that becomes overwhelming.

Developing a Search Strategy: Time as a Major Obstacle to Evidence-Based Practice

In my opinion, many articles and texts devoted to evidence-based practice and EBDM fail to truly acknowledge the real world of clinical practice. More often than not, they seem to be written by scholars for other scholars, that is, for people not frequently charged with daily clinical responsibilities. Yet busy clinicians at the "sharp end" of patient care are the intended target of the literature pertaining to evidence-based practice (**Figure 2.1**). The goal is to empower such clinicians with sound, evidence-based strategies, that is, to make evidence-based practice work at the grassroots level.

Nurse anesthetists are challenged in many ways in their professional lives, not the least of which is the time that they can devote to seeking evidence and searching the literature. Once a nurse anesthetist becomes cognizant of the principles of evidence-based practice and commits to being an evidence-based provider, I believe that time limitations

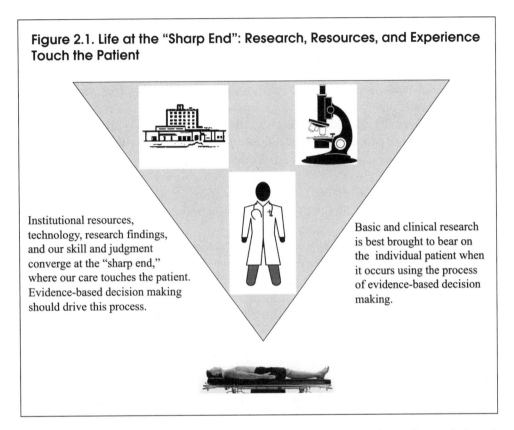

Figure 2.1. Life at the "Sharp End": Research, Resources, and Experience Touch the Patient

Institutional resources, technology, research findings, and our skill and judgment converge at the "sharp end," where our care touches the patient. Evidence-based decision making should drive this process.

Basic and clinical research is best brought to bear on the individual patient when it occurs using the process of evidence-based decision making.

represent the major obstacle to evidence-based practice. Given the realities of clinical care responsibility and time management, how is it best to proceed? Here are some practical illustrations of scenarios in which EBDM is warranted:

1. A student receives a clinical assignment the afternoon before the scheduled surgery and wants to select the best approach to managing a patient with cardiomyopathy-induced heart failure who is undergoing partial gastrectomy for a benign tumor. The patient is taking a β-blocker, an angiotensin-converting enzyme inhibitor, and has an indwelling central line for nutritional support with an intravenous fat emulsion (eg, Intralipid).

2. A Certified Registered Nurse Anesthetist (CRNA) comes to work and finds that he is assigned to the urology operating room. The second scheduled case is a radical open prostatectomy in an otherwise healthy 60-year-old man with insulin-controlled diabetes. The CRNA vaguely recalls having read an article on the use of preemptive ketamine that conveyed significant advantages intraoperatively and postoperatively for opiate conservation for analgesia.

3. Several weeks in advance, a staff CRNA is asked to present at the department's monthly case conference series on the use of atenolol for perioperative heart rate

control of patients with a history of coronary artery disease who are scheduled for noncardiac surgery. Although this approach is common in the institution, the CRNA is aware of recent research that challenges the routine use of β-blockers in this patient population.

4. A CRNA working in a children's hospital has extensive experience with the anesthetic management of patients undergoing the Nuss procedure (anterior thoracic wall bar placement for correction of pectus excavatum). The CRNA is unsatisfied with the usual course of postoperative pain control and wants to improve the outcome.

5. A CRNA with administrative responsibility for quality assurance finds a high rate of borderline to frank hypoxemia in adult patients on arrival to the PACU following general anesthesia. He observes a wide range of practice patterns with respect to patient transport from the operating room to the PACU and wants to develop some clinical practice guidelines.

6. A CRNA has an emergency case of appendicitis assigned to her, bumping the scheduled case to later in the day. A 67-year-old man with a long history of Charcot-Marie-Tooth disease arrives in the operating room, and the surgeon is pressing to start. Although she recalls taking care of a patient with Charcot-Marie-Tooth disease, she wants to refresh her knowledge and develop a plan of care.

In each case, the student or CRNA wants to engage in EBDM. The time and resource constraints associated with the scenarios vary considerably. Attempting to apply a singular approach to EBDM would be inappropriate, just as applying a singular approach to the anesthetic management of each of the patient scenarios would be inappropriate. Whether choosing a research design or an induction agent, or engaging in an evidence-based practice process, the context of the situation at hand is a major driving force in the decision how to proceed.

In scenarios 2 and 6, there are severe time constraints, and an extensive literature search will not be possible. In these situations, EBDM may hinge on the following:

- Discussing the case with an experienced and respected colleague
- Consulting an authoritative textbook
- Performing a quick electronic search of the literature

When there is a substantial time constraint, such as only 5 or 10 minutes to obtain the latest information from the literature, information from the National Center for Biotechnology Information (NCBI), the PubMed website, can be accessed. Established in 1988 as a national resource for molecular biology information, the NCBI now supports public databases, facilitates research in computational biology, and disseminates biomedical information to facilitate processes affecting human health and disease. This site has enormous applicability for nurse anesthetists when time is short.

Gaining the needed information and evidence for scenario 2 can be achieved by visiting the NCBI's PubMed website, http://www.PubMed.gov. On the NCBI website, the homepage lists PubMed services, including Journals Database, MeSH (Medical Subject Headings) Database, and others (**Figure 2.2**). Clicking on "Clinical Queries" leads to a new page entitled "PubMed Clinical Queries" where you can enter search terms. (In the example I use in Figure 2.2, the search terms include "tonsillectomy" and "dexamethasone" because many of us frequently employ this medication during this procedure.) Choosing "therapy" to focus your research is likely the most common clinical subject category that nurse anesthetists will be interested in. Once you enter your search terms, the PubMed tool will find relevant "papers" (articles) for you. Clicking on the title of

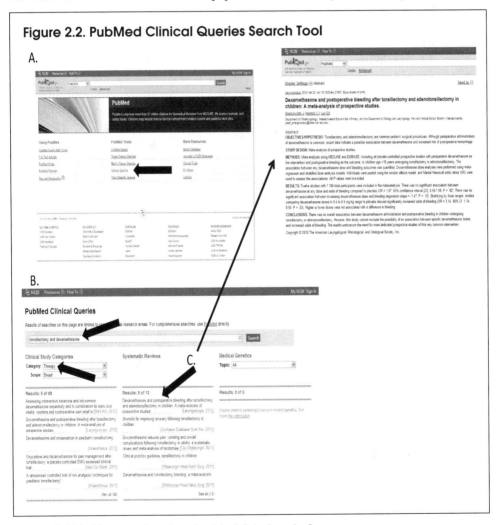

Figure 2.2. PubMed Clinical Queries Search Tool

A. Access PubMed @ www.pubmed.gov. Look for "clinical queries."

B. Enter your search terms here, eg, "Tonsillectomy and Dexamethasone" after choosing "Therapy" under the Clinical Study Categories offered by PubMed.

C. Click on a topic paper (here a metaanalysis that was found) to retrieve the synopsis.

(Reprinted with permission from the National Library of Medicine.)

interest (in Figure 2.2, I've selected a meta-analysis on the topic) will direct you to a synopsis of that paper. Abstracts of relevant trials as well as a list of related articles can be accessed as time permits. Using this rapid, specific search tool provides up-to-date information in a time-efficient manner.

More Extensive Searching of the Literature

The keys to EBDM are the latest and best information combined with experience and skill and including, as much as possible, the patient's desires and needs. **Figure 2.3** is a conceptual overview of evidence-based practice. Obtaining the necessary information can be the most time-consuming step in the process of evidence-based practice. In evidence-based practice, it is important to recognize that there comes a time when the benefits of continued searching may not be worth the effort required to identify more sources or publications. I conceptualize this step into what I call the "bull's-eye model" of evidence-based practice (**Figure 2.4**).

In any search for evidence relevant to a clinical question, a hierarchy of study designs and observations will be encountered (**Figure 2.5**). Many factors and issues related to study design, publication bias (tendency to favor research with positive findings), author editorialization, statistical treatment, sample size, placebo effects, and other elements can hamper attempts to interpret the literature.

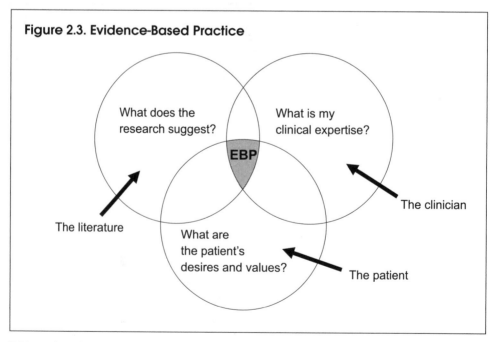

Figure 2.3. Evidence-Based Practice

What does the research suggest?

What is my clinical expertise?

EBP

The literature

The clinician

What are the patient's desires and values?

The patient

Evidence-based practice (EBP) occurs at the intersection of the literature, the clinician, and the patient and is thus highly context sensitive.

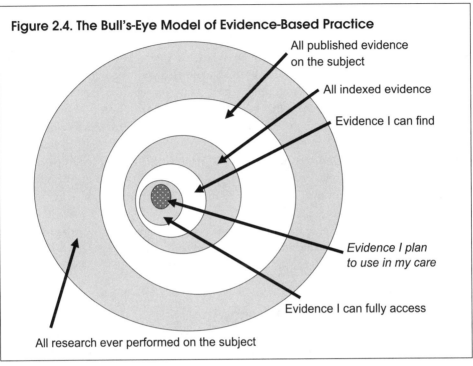

Figure 2.4. The Bull's-Eye Model of Evidence-Based Practice

All published evidence on the subject

All indexed evidence

Evidence I can find

Evidence I plan to use in my care

Evidence I can fully access

All research ever performed on the subject

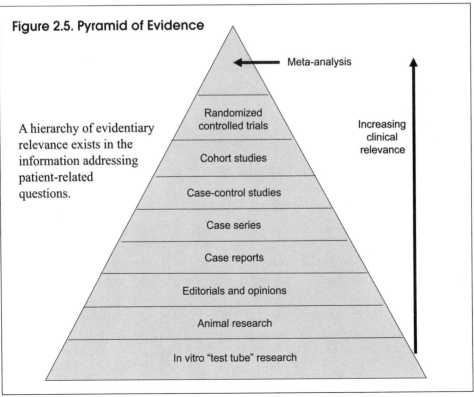

Figure 2.5. Pyramid of Evidence

Meta-analysis

A hierarchy of evidentiary relevance exists in the information addressing patient-related questions.

Increasing clinical relevance

Randomized controlled trials

Cohort studies

Case-control studies

Case series

Case reports

Editorials and opinions

Animal research

In vitro "test tube" research

An example is the "N-of-1 randomized controlled trial (RCT)." In this type of trial, a single patient participates in pairs of treatment periods in which one interventional treatment is given in one period and a placebo or alternative intervention is given in the other period. Neither the patient nor the clinician has knowledge of the intervention, and the intervention order is controlled and randomized. This type of study continues until the patient and the clinician conclude that benefit or failure has resulted. The N-of-1 RCT is not appropriate in a number of circumstances, such as short-duration problems, surgical care, and interventions that require many months (or years) to play out. In this type of 1-patient, crossover trial, specific information is obtained for the particular patient generally in the setting of clinical practice. Thus, it is not generalizable to other patients but can have great merit in evaluating a new treatment (compared with an older one) in a specific patient.

Large clinical studies require generalization of results observed in study participants to a specific patient, a process that invariably leads to some degree of research-to-practice chasm. That chasm can be bridged somewhat by selectiveness in the level of research used in the decision-making process.

The 4S Mnemonic as an Efficiency Tool

A literature search for the most relevant evidence should not focus on books as the primary information source for a variety of reasons (eg, possibly substantial bias, possibly dated material, risk of misinterpreting primary reference sources, and uncertainty about chapter authorship decisions). When possible, the focus should include the following:

- Primary studies: highly relevant study designs that minimize bias and have strong internal validity
- Summaries: systematic reviews with a strong methodology that critically overviews the existing evidence
- Synopses: brief encapsulations of individual studies or systematic reviews that provide key points about methods, results, and conclusions
- Systematic consensus guidelines and advisories: evidence-based clinical pathways or summaries in a targeted domain that help guide decision making

The preceding classification is the "4S" scheme, based on studies, summaries, synopses, and systematic domain-targeted guidelines. Such an approach will help busy clinicians keep pace with the necessary but expanding rate of evidence accumulation.

Evolving alongside the EBDM movement, which has occurred worldwide, has been the proliferation of electronic search tools and secondary journals devoted to facilitating access to the world's literature. Although I have not precisely counted the number of electronic bibliographic databases available, worldwide, these number in the hundreds. What makes these electronic-based search and access tools so useful to clinicians is their unparalleled ability to use the latest technologies in expeditiously matching patient-related attributes and patient-related problems with the most relevant and valid research evidence. Appendix 2.1 lists my favorite websites. For a more comprehensive list of electronic search tools, see the Appendix at the end of the book.

Based on the 4S mnemonic, citations are restricted exclusively to studies of excellent design and that provide most, if not all, of the clinical and basic research information needed for EBDM. In particular, the high-quality, systematic review databases available through sites such as The Cochrane Collaboration are designed to provide an ever-expanding repository of valid and practical clinical summaries. Because of the importance and particular historical and contemporary relevance of The Cochrane Collaboration, Chapter 8 is devoted to its history, access, and use.

Evaluating the Information Retrieved

A critical step in the EBDM process is evaluating, in the context of the patient or patient group under immediate consideration, the worth and applicability of the retrieved studies. Nurse anesthesia programs have increasingly emphasized the preparation of practitioners with excellent critical reading and evaluation skills, and for good reason. Referring again to Figure 2.4, it is obvious that a filtering effect takes place in the EBDM process. Study selection is followed by further assessment (with attention to internal and external validity), followed by their further analysis in the specific context of the patient or patients under consideration.

The following are general, all-purpose questions to consider when evaluating research articles for the EBDM process. See Appendix 2.2 for a comprehensive checklist.

1. Does the study address a clinically relevant and focused question?
2. Is the study internally valid (randomization, subject/observer blinding, methods exacting and well controlled)?
3. Do the patients in the study "look like" the patients you care for (external validity)?
4. Are the relevant outcomes captured in a valid and reliable way?
5. Have baseline group attributes been accounted for, measured, and balanced so that known (and even unknown) moderating factors have been controlled for?
6. Are the statistical methods sufficiently described and appropriate?
7. Is the sample size adequate to properly empower the statistical procedures used?
8. If subjects dropped out of the study or were otherwise lost from the analysis, have the researchers explained why?
9. Did the researchers stick to the focused question or hypothesis and avoid editorializing beyond the boundaries of the research design?

The bottom line in evaluating studies is determining their worth and applicability to the patients receiving care. The ability to evaluate is a complex undertaking at the upper end of cognitive ability (**Figure 2.6**)[4]. A CRNA's ability to critically evaluate and interpret studies and evaluate their worth is vital to the EBDM process.

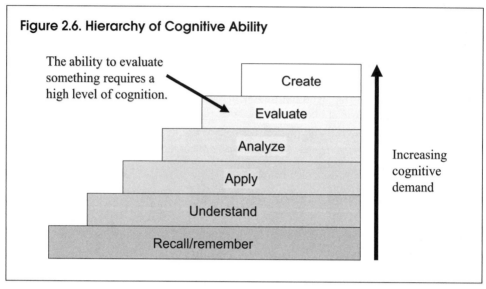

Figure 2.6. Hierarchy of Cognitive Ability

The ability to evaluate something requires a high level of cognition.

Create

Evaluate

Analyze

Apply

Understand

Recall/remember

Increasing cognitive demand

(Based on Bloom et al.[4])

Levels of Evidence and Levels of Recommendations

A number of evaluatory and rating systems have been developed and are referred to on many of the evidence-based practice websites and search tools. Two examples reflecting this type of research hierarchy are endorsed by the Agency for Healthcare Research and Quality and the US Preventive Services Task Force for ranking the strength of evidence related to the effectiveness of an intervention.

In England, the National Health Service uses a similar categorical system; the following levels are applicable to treatments and other medical and nursing interventions:

- Level A: consistent randomized controlled trial, cohort study
- Level B: consistent retrospective cohort, exploratory cohort, epidemiologic study, outcomes research, case-control study, or extrapolations from level A studies
- Level C: case-series study or extrapolations from level B studies
- Level D: expert opinion without explicit critical appraisal or based on physiology, bench research, or accepted scientific principles

Although the language may confuse some American readers and despite the semantic differences between the American and English classifications, the intended goal is to assist users of clinical research to use the findings of studies that are most likely to be valid. Nevertheless, the ultimate decision to use the findings of a particular study rests with the clinician, highlighting the need to thoughtfully engage in critical appraisal.

I find that practical guidelines directed at clinicians are most often of greatest practical use. The US Preventive Services Task Force grading (**Table 2.2**) uses a set of levels for

Table 2.2. Commonly Cited Scales Reflecting Levels of Evidence

Categories of Research: Evidence Hierarchies	
Level I	Meta-analysis (combination of data from many studies)
Level II	Experimental designs (randomized controlled trials)
Level III	Well-designed, quasi-experimental designs (not randomized or no control group)
Level IV	Well-designed nonexperimental designs (descriptive, can include qualitative)
Level V	Case reports/clinical expertise

Relevance and Usefulness of the Evidence	
A	Strongly recommended; good evidence
B	Recommended; at least fair evidence
C	No recommendation; balance of benefits and harms too close to justify a recommendation
D	Recommend against; fair evidence is ineffective or harm outweighs the benefit
I	Insufficient evidence; evidence is lacking or of poor quality, benefit and harms cannot be determined

(Adapted from Agency for Healthcare Research and Quality.[5])

its guidelines for a clinical intervention.[4] Here, the focus is on a risk-benefit ratio of the intervention in combination with the level of evidence on which the recommendation is based. To elaborate, this classification scheme is based on the following:

- Level A: Good scientific evidence suggests that the benefits of the clinical service substantially outweigh the potential risks. Clinicians should discuss the service with eligible patients.
- Level B: At least fair scientific evidence suggests that the benefits of the clinical service outweigh the potential risks. Clinicians should discuss the service with eligible patients.
- Level C: At least fair scientific evidence suggests that there are benefits provided by the clinical service, but the balance between benefits and risks is too close for making general recommendations. Clinicians need not offer it unless there are individual considerations.

- Level D: At least fair scientific evidence suggests that the risks of the clinical service outweigh potential benefits. Clinicians should not routinely offer the service to asymptomatic patients.
- Level I: Scientific evidence is lacking, of poor quality, or conflicting, such that the risk vs benefit balance cannot be assessed. Clinicians should help patients understand the uncertainty surrounding the clinical service.

These evidentiary rankings are useful to clinicians because they provide yet another perspective in judging the worth of research to assist in EBDM for a patient or focused group of patients.

Implementing the Plan in the Context of the Patient or Patient Population, Based on the Evidence

There are limitations to unsystematically obtained clinical observations, even when they may be based on classic, well-accepted physiological rationale. We can look back at some examples that were clearly and, occasionally, even catastrophically, incorrect:

- The use of growth hormone in critically ill patients[6]
- Combining certain vasodilators and inotropic agents in patients with heart failure[7]
- Use of β-carotene in patients with prior myocardial infarction[8]
- Use of inhaled nitric oxide in respiratory distress due to hypoxia or asthma[9]
- Hormone therapy to reduce cardiovascular disease risk reduction in women[9]
- IgM monoclonal antibody therapy to treat gram-negative sepsis[9]

Certainly, it can be argued that any empirical observation made between an intervention and a result constitutes a form of evidence, even when the observation is made unsystematically. Of course, such observations are prone to a variety of limitations that are discussed throughout this text. These limitations focus back on the hierarchy of evidence referred to earlier (see Figure 2.5). When it comes to implementing a plan, the plan should be based on the very best evidence, in the context of the unique patient circumstances. What guidelines should be followed?

A given intervention is not likely to be effective in every patient. No matter what body of evidence used in the EBDM process, it is important to recognize that findings are being generalized from results achieved with patients other than the patients we encounter in our clinical work. Furthermore, even the hierarchical nature of the evidence pyramid can fail us. As we shall see in Chapter 3, a lower level of evidence, such as that from an observational study, can often provide more compellingly applicable, real-world information than the randomized trial can.

Evidence-Based Decision Making Is More Than Just Research Reports

Often underemphasized in a discussion of evidence-based practice is the essential value of clinical experience and clinical judgment, as well as an understanding of individual patients in the context of their personality, culture, and unique experiences. Even with a substantial amount of meaningful evidence to apply, a lack of experience and judgment may result in enormous faltering in its application to individual patients. Experience and judgment are indispensable when considering and ranking interventional options. Certainly, part of the EBDM process is based on consideration of the skill of the clinicians in the studies selected to evaluate and whether all important outcomes have been measured. Similarly, sensitivity to a patient's desires and beliefs is vitally important in taking full advantage of an evidence-based practice approach to care.

Most of EBDM related to anesthesia care is played out in circumstances in which the patient's input is likely to be minimal to nonexistent (eg, choice of neuromuscular blocking drug, intraoperative fluid management, selection of antifibrinolytic, approach to managing body temperature and its measurement, and type and settings of ventilator management). However, many decisions should actively involve patients, especially of risk-benefit issues (eg, regional vs general anesthesia, perioperative blood transfusion, postoperative nausea and pain control, and management of the risks of vision disturbances and peripheral nerve injury).

Although a goal of evidence-based practice is to provide the best care possible in the unique contextual situation of a given patient, another is for nurse anesthetists to act as patient advocates. Basing our interventions on the triad of the latest research evidence, our clinical expertise and experience, and the needs and wishes of the patient (see Figure 2.3) requires CRNAs to act as patient advocates throughout the process. Evidence-based practice is, by definition, the marriage of excellent clinical science with humanitarian consideration of patients as people. Extracting the contextually essential, best information from the vast, representative research literature and merging it with the art of applying it to a patient is evidence-based practice at its finest.

As the initial recommendation to ask the right question is revisited and preparation is made to apply the intervention to the patient, the following questions must be asked:

- Is the patient well represented by the studies selected?
- Is the planned intervention one with which we are familiar and experienced?
- What are the risks of the intervention; does gain outpace the drawbacks?
- When possible, has the patient been adequately informed and drawn into the decision-making process?

With satisfactory responses to each of the questions, the intervention or interventions can be applied. Next, it is time to evaluate the outcome of the intervention.

Evaluating the Intervention

As stated earlier and illustrated in Figure 2.6, evaluation is an extremely complex cognitive function.[4] By definition, to *evaluate* something is to determine how useful or valuable something is, judging its suitability by predetermined criteria. The criteria likely to be considered in evaluating a planned intervention include the following, among possible others:

- Cost (money, time expenditure, associated equipment needs)
- Feasibility to perform in the individual clinical setting
- Ease (or difficulty) of technique
- Patient's likely length of stay (eg, in the operating room, PACU, or hospital)
- Patient function
- Patient quality of life
- Demonstrated risks of morbidity (eg, harm and associated complications)
- Demonstrated risk of mortality
- Potential for unplanned readmission
- Assessment of overall benefit

Intraoperative Glucose Control, Use of Perioperative β-Blockers, and a Word to the Wise

Examples of the application of evidence-based decision making abound, and the necessity of an ongoing process of evaluation is essential. Areas of considerable recent and ongoing controversy concern the intraoperative control of glucose levels and the use of β-blockers in patients deemed at risk of cardiovascular events. Although hyperglycemia can clearly be harmful, the current status of clinical evidence does not urge the routine use of "tight glycemic control" in which the patient's blood glucose level is targeted at 80 to 110 mg/dL. A compelling trial published in 2001 revealed significant advantages when such control was achieved in a large group of surgical intensive care unit patients.[10] Decreased mortality, decreased morbidity, and reduction in bloodstream infections were found. A follow-up study has shed a somewhat different light on the domain, noting that these findings may not apply at all to patients in the medical intensive care unit.[11] Other studies were stopped prematurely because of safety concerns,[12,13] with yet another trial demonstrating an increase in stroke and death with tight glycemic control in cardiac surgery patients.[14] At this time, the efficacy and safety of tight glycemic control await further evidence before consensus guidelines can be recommended. A recent, evidence-based review of the subject underscores these concerns and notes the frequent inherent difficulty in categorizing and operationalizing measures of quality in the care provided to patients.[15]

Another area of contentious debate awaiting further evidence is the perioperative use of β-blockers to avoid poor outcomes in patients at risk of cardiovascular events. The POISE trial (PeriOperative ISchemic Evaluation trial) revealed a reduction of myocardial infarction.[16,17] (However, a large proportion of the diagnoses were made in patients without overt signs and were based on electrocardiographic or enzyme changes, with few cases resulting in the development of congestive cardiac failure, the need for emergency repeated interventional surgery, or nonfatal arrests.[16,17]) The flip side of the largest randomized trial of its kind was the finding that the incidence of stroke, overall patient disability, and mortality was increased in patients receiving β-blockers.[17] Although the POISE trial has been widely criticized, it has given us pause, and, as is so often the case, we must await further evidence to illuminate the correct path for individual patient decision making.

Although systematic evaluation of an intervention's outcome is traditionally the terrain of clinical researchers, participating in and completing the process of evidence-based practice necessitates that practitioners evaluate, to the best of their ability, the intervention performed. The bottom line is that if we perform an intervention, in this case an evidence-based intervention, we want to know its effect or effects on the patient in terms of benefit, harm, cost, and feasibility.

References

1. McGlynn EA, Asch SM, Adams J, et al. The quality of health care delivered to adults in the United States. *N Engl J Med.* 2003;348(26):2635-2645.

2. Committee on Quality of Health Care in America, Institute of Medicine. *Crossing the Quality Chasm: A New Health System for the 21st Century.* Washington, DC: National Academies Press; 2001.

3. Druss BG, Marcus SC, Offson M, Tanielian T, Elinson L, Pincus HA. Comparing the national economic burden of 5 chronic conditions. *Health Aff.* 2001;20(6):233-241.

4. Bloom B, Englehart M, Furst E, Hill W, Krathwohl D. The classification of educational goals. In: Bloom BS, ed. *Taxonomy of Educational Objectives Handbook I: Cognitive Domain.* New York, NY: Longman; 1956.

5. Agency for Healthcare Research and Quality. US Preventive Services Task Force ratings: grade definitions. *Guide to Clinical Preventive Services, Third Edition: Periodic Updates, 2000-2003.* http://www.ahrq.gov/clinic/3rduspstf/ratings.htm. Accessed September 11, 2012.

6. Takala J, Ruokomen E, Webster NR, et al. Increased mortality associated with growth hormone treatment in critically ill adults. *N Engl J Med.* 1999;341(11):785-792.

7. Hamton JR, van Veldhuisen DJ, Kleber FX, et al. Randomised study of effect of ibopamine on survival in patients with advanced severe heart failure. *Lancet.* 1997;349(9057):971-977.

8. Rapola JM, Virtamo J, Ripatti S, et al. Randomised trial of alpha-tocopherol and beta-carotene supplements on incidents of major coronary events in men with previous infarction. *Lancet.* 1997;349(9067):1715-1720.

9. Ioannidis JPA. Contradicted and initially stronger effects in highly cited clinical research. *JAMA*. 2005;294(2):218-228.

10. Van den Berghe G, Wouters P, Weekers F, et al. Intensive insulin therapy in critically ill patients. *N Engl J Med*. 2001;345(19):1359-1367.

11. Van den Berghe G, Wilmer A, Hermans G. Intensive insulin therapy in the medical ICU. *N Engl J Med*. 2006;354(5):449-461.

12. Brunkhorst FM, Engel C, Bloos F, et al; for German Competence Network Sepsis (SepNet). Intensive insulin therapy and pentastarch resuscitation in severe sepsis. *N Engl J Med*. 2008;358(2):125-139.

13. Preiser JC. Restoring normoglycaemia: not so harmless [editorial]. *Crit Care*. 2008;12(1):116.

14. Gandhi GY, Nuttall GA, Abel MD, et al. Intensive intraoperative insulin therapy versus conventional glucose management during cardiac surgery: a randomized trial. *Ann Intern Med*. 2007;146(4):233-243.

15. Lipshutz AK, Gropper MA. Perioperative glycemic control: an evidence-based review. *Anesthesiology*. 2009;110(2):408-421.

16. POISE Trial Investigators, Devereaux PJ, Yang H, et al. Rationale, design, and organization of the PeriOperative ISchemic Evaluation (POISE) trial: a randomized controlled trial of metoprolol versus placebo in patients undergoing noncardiac surgery. *Am Heart J*. 2006;52(2):223-230.

17. POISE Study Group, Devereaux PJ, Yang H, et al. Effects of extended-release metoprolol succinate in patients undergoing non-cardiac surgery (POISE trial): a randomised controlled trial. *Lancet*. 2008;371(9627):1839-1847.

Appendix 2.1. Exemplary Websites of Relevance and Worth in Accessing the Literature

The following is a list of websites that I have found to be readily accessible and easy to use. The list is far from comprehensive.

ACP (American College of Physicians) Journal Club
http://acpjc.acponline.org

Bandolier
http://www.medicine.ox.ac.uk/bandolier

The Cochrane Collaboration and Library
http://www.cochrane.org

Centre for Evidence-based Medicine (University of Oxford)
http://www.cebm.net

Essential Evidence Plus
http://www.essentialevidenceplus.com

Evidence-Based Perioperative Medicine
http://www.ebpom.org/publications

General resource information
http://www.dartmouth.edu/~biomed/resources.htmld/guides/ebmresources.shtml

MEDLINE, US National Library of Medicine
http://www.nlm.nih.gov/databases/databases_medline.html

National Guideline Clearinghouse
http://www.guidelines.gov

Ovid
http://www.ovid.com

PubMed Clinical Queries
http://www.ncbi.nlm.nih.gov/pubmed/clinical

Appendix 2.2. A Checklist for Evaluation of Individual Research Articles

This checklist proposes a systematic manner to help determine the merit and validity of a clinical research report for potential clinical application.

√ Introduction

Does it address an appropriate and clearly focused question or hypothesis?
Is sufficient, up-to-date information presented to justify the study's purpose?
Is the population to which the investigators intend to refer their findings identified?

√ Design of the study

Is it an experiment, a planned observation, or an analysis of records?
Is it a representative, well-defined sample? Is the sample biased in some way?
Is the intervention to be tested justified and well described?
Are the attributes of the control and comparison groups well described?
Are the definitions of terms clear throughout, including the outcome measures?
Are potentially confounding variables and factors accounted for and controlled in some way?
Are outcome measures collected in a standardized, valid, and reliable way?
Are statistical procedures appropriate to the nature of the data and properly performed?

√ Presentation of findings

Are the findings presented clearly, objectively, and in sufficient detail?
Are there any issues related to statistical versus clinical significance? If so, are they discussed?
Are numbers and reasons for dropouts and/or missing data described?

√ Conclusions

Are the conclusions relevant to the original question, objective, or hypothesis?
Are the conclusions justified by the findings? Which are not?
Does the discussion section incorporate relevant research as it relates to the current study?
What (if any) are the implications and relevance to clinical practice?

CHAPTER THREE

Randomized Controlled Trials and Nonrandomized Observational Studies

Although it is impossible to forecast future theoretical and practical advances in research methods, of the methods currently available, the randomized controlled trial (RCT) is the optimal method for measuring the effect or effects of a clinical intervention in a particular setting. As shown in Chapter 2 in the discussion of the hierarchical nature of research (see Figure 2.5), the RCT is subordinate only to the meta-analysis, which is explored in greater detail in Chapter 7. Briefly, a meta-analysis is a collection of RCTs meeting specific criteria that have been combined, using a common metric and special statistical methods, to provide a pooled estimate of the effects of the intervention or interventions under study.

In an RCT, research subjects are randomly assigned, or "randomized," to various "arms" of the study. One arm is usually a control group. The control group might receive a placebo or sham intervention, or it might receive the current "gold standard" intervention. Another arm of the study might involve a new or hybridized intervention. An RCT may have several arms, allowing for multiple interventions to be compared in a single trial or for the same intervention to be tested in several magnitudes. The latter is typical of trials involving drugs, in which different dosages are applied to gauge efficacy, the side-effect profile, and safety. Randomization reduces bias by rendering treatment and control groups equivalent with respect to known and unknown confounders. If an adequate sample size is obtained and appropriate statistical procedures are applied, randomization can help determine if any observed differences in outcome are due to a particular intervention. Furthermore, RCTs allow researchers to make relatively confident assessments regarding cause-and-effect relationships, something that is not possible with retrospective methods.

Figure 3.1 illustrates a fictional trial comparing 3 antifibrinolytic agents used in cardiac surgery to reduce the need for transfusion. The starting group of 21 open-heart surgical patients is randomized to receive antifibrinolytic A, B, or C. The patients undergo anesthesia and surgery and the antifibrinolytic intervention. They are then followed up for 90 days, with the primary outcome measures being survival and number of units of blood transfused perioperatively. Group differences in mortality would be assessed with a nonparametric procedure such as the χ^2 test, and group differences in

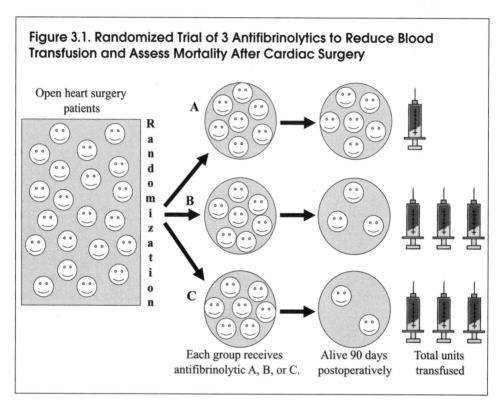

Figure 3.1. Randomized Trial of 3 Antifibrinolytics to Reduce Blood Transfusion and Assess Mortality After Cardiac Surgery

the amount of blood transfused would be assessed with a parametric tool such as the analysis of variance. Using a tool that allows the computation of a measure such as the relative risk or the odds ratio would allow quantification of the magnitude of the effect of interventions A, B, and C on the outcomes of interest. (See Chapter 5 for discussion of effect size measures.)

The concept of *external validity* is an important one that is often inadequately considered by researchers and clinician-consumers alike. External validity deals with the issue of generalizability—to whom can the findings of the study be applied? In the effort to achieve as much control as possible over potentially influencing factors, RCTs are often restricted to patients with limited comorbidity and include patients taking as few medications as possible. This approach is clearly rational from the researcher's perspective, whose goal is to ascertain, as rigorously as possible, the effect of an intervention (eg, use of atenolol perioperatively) on an outcome (eg, perioperative myocardial infarction). For instance, a study that includes 55- to 70-year old men with hypertension controlled by angiotensin-converting enzyme inhibitors who are randomized to perioperatively receive placebo or atenolol and who are undergoing hip arthroplasty under spinal anesthesia provides the researcher with powerful experimental control, but equally powerful limitations. Internal validity and experimental rigor may be high, but women, people with diabetes, men not in the 55- to 70-year age group, patients having general anesthesia, and patients undergoing procedures other than hip arthroplasty will not benefit from such a study. In this example, external validity would be absent for patients who differ in characteristics from the study subjects.

A factor often not considered is that patients entering an RCT may differ from patients at large because they are agreeable to being part of an experimental process. In some cases, the study design may involve the risk of assignment to a placebo treatment or to a therapy with an effect that is poorly described or even associated with major complications. Although it is difficult to appreciate the importance (if any) of such a difference in patient psychological attributes, this difference is an example of a potentially confounding factor. Consider for yourself: if you had a serious medical condition and were asked to enroll in an RCT evaluating a promising new therapy, one arm of which was a placebo group, would you participate, given the potential to be randomized to the placebo group?

Efficacy and Effectiveness: Nonequivalent Terms!

An RCT generally demonstrates *efficacy* rather than *effectiveness*, terms that many use interchangeably but that have markedly different associations. *Efficacy* is the treatment effect under the highly (artificially) controlled conditions of the RCT and refers to whether an intervention produces the expected result under ideal circumstances. *Effectiveness* is the treatment effect under the conditions of usual, real-world practice and represents a more pragmatic consideration of the magnitude of benefit under real-world conditions. Thus, the concept of effectiveness is more reflective of what is likely to be observed in patients encountered on an everyday basis.

There are times when RCTs are simply unavailable for consideration and for many reasons, including issues related to expense, time, risk, and ethics. In such cases, nonrandomized, observational studies (NROS) represent reasonable alternatives to RCTs to quantify effectiveness and other real-world outcomes. An example is the evaluation of drug-eluting stents, interventions receiving substantial attention not only in medical and nursing journals but also in the lay press. The RCTs of stents have demonstrated short-term efficacy for relatively healthy patients, and NROS are revealing questionable long-term effectiveness and safety problems in a much broader range of patients.[1] It was just such an observational study that caused researchers to reexamine the use of the antifibrinolytic agent aprotinin, which ultimately led to its abandonment because of excessive rates of renal failure, heart failure, myocardial infarction, and serious cerebral events in the patients who received it.[2] Phase 4 trials, also referred to as postmarketing surveillance trials, are examples of the NROS.

Consider the highly publicized case of rofecoxib (Vioxx), a drug that was removed from the market in 2004 in the wake of a maelstrom of incriminating evidence after observational research findings revealed it to be associated with an accelerated risk of heart attack, thrombosis, stroke, and death, likely due to its downstream effect on increasing thromboxane levels in users.[3] Thromboxane is a special lipid (an eicosanoid) that is produced in platelets; its 2 forms, A2 and B2, encourage platelet clumping and blood vessel constriction.

Although observational data are not randomized and they lack many elements of prospective, interventional control, there are many acceptable approaches for making statistical inferences from such data. Because observational studies lack control for selection and assignment biases, special statistical methods involving matching, stratification, and/or covariance adjustment are needed.

In the NROS, the researcher identifies outcomes that are scientifically related to the intervention that was applied. The issue, of course, is that in such a study, the patients have not been randomized to the respective interventions. Such studies require careful analysis to put them in proper perspective. The goal of the analytical tools that focus on observational data is to create an analysis that resembles what would occur if the treatment had been randomly assigned. (See "Use of Propensity Score Analysis" later in this chapter.) A critical reader may ask whether such an assumption is reasonable. This rather lofty goal is one that study designers hope for but do not always achieve. The task of the readers of the research report is to decipher the credibility of the reported findings. Credibility is not something that can consistently be counted on, and my advice is to be cautious when reading the conclusions of authors who rely on observational techniques, especially if they claim cause-and-effect relationships. Nevertheless, such studies can reveal clinically relevant associations (as with aprotinin, rofecoxib, droperidol, and others) that set the stage for more stringently conducted subsequent research, such as an RCT.

Essential Differences Between the RCT and NROS

There are fundamental differences between the RCT and the NROS. In an RCT, one goal is to balance study participant characteristics present before the treatment is administered. The success of randomization in creating balance can be assessed even before treatment interventions are applied. Researchers describe the attributes (demographics) of the treatment groups in their research reports—a fundamental requirement for publication. Whether presented in the text or in a table, readers can determine whether the characteristics of subjects in the arms of the study are equally distributed. This information is helpful in several ways. For one, it helps determine whether patients in the study have characteristics similar to those of the patients encountered in clinical practice, an essential question in any evidence-based inquiry. Second, it helps readers assess the representative balance of patient characteristics that might influence the outcome. Relevant patient characteristics vary considerably from study to study; common ones are listed in **Table 3.1**.

In an NROS, a primary goal is to use statistical techniques that create balance between treatments or characteristics that are assessed before the actual treatment or intervention is applied. If this balance is satisfactorily achieved, the outcome can be measured and comparisons made between or among groups. This objective may be difficult to achieve for a number of reasons. For example, there may be unmeasured, poorly measured, or unknown characteristics. This issue can be of great concern to readers who may, on their own, think of factors that constitute confounders of the relationships measured yet see no evidence that the researchers considered these confounders.

> **Table 3.1. Examples of Demographic Information**
>
> Gender
> Age
> ASA physical status
> Body habitus, height, and weight
> Medications
> Comorbidities
> Type of surgery
> Laboratory data (eg, preoperative hemoglobin and potassium levels)
> Vital signs
> Baseline exercise tolerance
> Cigarette smoking history

Relevant information about patient characteristics will vary considerably depending on the goals of a particular study. Ensuring equivalent representation between or among treatment arms helps control for unintended bias. As described in the text, there may be unknown (or unknowable) confounders that are not accounted for.

To adjust for pretreatment imbalances, 2 statistical approaches often used are analysis of covariance methods and propensity score analysis. These 2 methods complement each other and generally should be used together rather than using one or the other alone.

Use of Propensity Score Analysis

Consider an institution in which there is variation in technique for central line placement and one that has a good database allowing identification of preprocedural patient factors. This database also includes reliable documentation of complications and successful insertions associated with the techniques used. An observational study is performed involving ultrasound-guided central line placement vs central line placement using superficial anatomical landmarks. The goal is to estimate the effectiveness and safety of the 2 approaches by comparing preselected outcomes (eg, speed of placement and complication rates) for patients who were not randomly assigned to the interventions. A preintervention covariate (such as gender, age, use of a particular medication, or presence of a comorbidity) is selected that was unaffected by the intervention. In an RCT, such covariates would be expected to be balanced in distribution between the groups so that confounders would exert their effect equivalently on each arm of the study. In an NROS, the propensity score represents a way for researchers to construct matched pairs or stratifications that balance observed covariates. The propensity score for an individual is the probability of having been treated based on the individual's background (pretreatment) characteristics. Intuitively, the propensity score is a measure of the likelihood that a person would have been treated based on his or her background characteristics had the study, in fact, been an RCT.

Mathematically the propensity score is simply the probability (between 0 and 1) that a participant is in the treated group vs the control group, given his or her background (pretreatment) characteristics. Think of it this way: The propensity score is usually estimated by using logistic regression, in which the treatment variable is the outcome, and the background characteristics, not the study outcomes, are the predictor variables in the model. Further discussion of the propensity score is provided in an excellent overview by Joffe and Rosenbaum.[4]

Propensity score modeling should be assessed, as would randomization in an RCT, on its performance in creating balance and not on the basis of the eventual treatment-effect estimates. The decision about whether a propensity score model "worked" should be made based only on examining the characteristics measured on participants before the collection of any outcome measures. Propensity score analysis is increasingly being presented in articles that find their way into the anesthesia and critical care literature.

Final Considerations

The RCT is generally considered the gold standard in biomedical research but often cannot be performed for a variety of reasons. In an NROS, patients and providers self-select for receiving the treatment or not receiving it, which may limit interpretation primarily because of loss of control over influencing factors and the real potential of bias. However, even in an RCT, there is a form of self-selection operative in the study population. My colleague, an oncologist at the University of Florida, and I have detailed our concerns about this issue previously in *JAMA* and in a journal devoted to cancer research.[5,6] For example, patients who decide to allow themselves to be randomized to receive a treatment (eg, an investigational drug that promotes tissue oxygen diffusion in critically ill, anesthetized patients) are not necessarily a random sample of all potential patients. In fact, in many cases, RCTs have inclusion and exclusion criteria that are so stringently restrictive that participants are unlikely to be fully representative of people who may ultimately receive the treatment once it becomes available. In general, data emerging from an NROS more closely resemble patients that we care for in the highly heterogeneous world of daily practice.

Ideally, studies would include all people who might benefit from the intervention under consideration, not just a subset of people comfortable with being randomized to receive a treatment and who fit the particular inclusion and exclusion criteria of a given trial. Conducting clinical research is akin to keeping a balance between "control over variables" and "application to patients at large." Like a child's playground seesaw, too heavily favoring one side shifts the balance predictably (**Figure 3.2**).

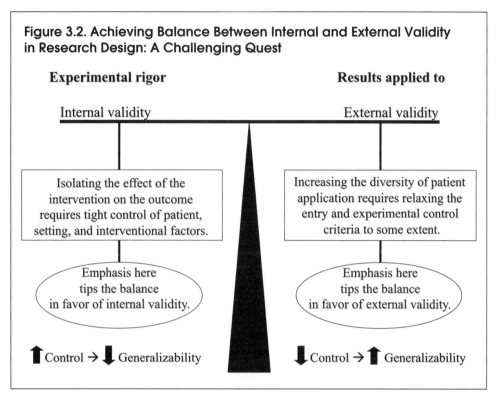

Figure 3.2. Achieving Balance Between Internal and External Validity in Research Design: A Challenging Quest

Symbols - Up arrow, increased; down arrow, decreased.

References

1. Eisenstein EI, Anstrom, KJ, Kong DF, et al. Clopidogrel use and long-term clinical outcomes after drug-eluting stent implantation. *JAMA.* 2007;297(2):159-168.

2. Mangano DT, Tudor JC, Dietzel C; for Multicenter Study of Perioperative Ischemia Research Group and the Ischemia Research and Education Foundation. The risk associated with aprotinin in cardiac surgery. *N Engl J Med.* 2006;354(4):353-365.

3. Mukherjee D, Nissen SE, Topol EJ. Risk of cardiovascular events associated with selective COX-2 inhibitors. *JAMA.* 2001;286(8):954-959.

4. Joffe MM, Rosenbaum PR. Invited commentary: propensity scores. *Am J Epidemiol.* 1999;150(4):327-333.

5. Amdur R, Biddle C. Institutional review board approval and publication of human research results. *JAMA.* 1997;277(11):909-914.

6. Amdur R, Biddle C. An algorithm for evaluating the ethics of a placebo-controlled trial. *Int J Cancer.* 2001;96(5):261-269.

CHAPTER FOUR

Voyages in Translational Research and Gauging Its Importance

Many fascinating stories exemplify bench-to-bedside research, a domain now referred to as translational research. Consider the discovery of warfarin as a deadly moisture-promoted pollutant in the feed of dairy cows and its eventual use to save the life of President Dwight D. Eisenhower. Imagine what the early experiments performed by Philip Drinker must have been like as he ushered in the birth of the iron lung to save victims of polio. Selman Waksman's discovery of streptomycin after isolating the producing fungus from the respiratory tract of a chicken was surrounded by the drama associated with a burgeoning infectious disease epidemic of tuberculosis. Envision Charles Waterton's classic experiments in 1825 in which he kept a donkey, to which he had given curare, alive by artificial ventilation, ultimately leading Harold Griffith and Enid Johnson to administer this substance to a surgical patient in 1942. The success of deep-brain stimulation for treating the symptoms of Parkinson disease was the result of decades of animal research into the basic anatomy and connectivity of the brain and the pathology of neurologic disorders.

Think back to the time of the discovery of cortisone, which occurred at the Mayo Clinic in the mid-20th century. A research biochemist isolated a material from the adrenal gland that was believed to harbor therapeutic promise. An established drug manufacturing company synthesized and made available enough of the material to allow Mayo Clinic clinician-scientists to design and perform a clinical trial in patients with rheumatoid arthritis. Interestingly enough, this occurred before healthcare research and development became an area of potential financial bonanza, and no economic reward was accorded the Mayo Clinic, only the advancement of science for the benefit of patients. Basic science translated into clinical application for the singular goal of improving the lives of patients. The list of bench-to-bedside voyages is as extensive as the interventions that we use for patients every day.

What is translational research? Its most utilitarian definition for our purposes is that it is the harnessing of knowledge gleaned from basic science research to produce interventions that are used in patients. Although variations of the definition abound, the importance of translational research is well appreciated. In fact, the National Institutes of Health has made this type of research a priority, forming centers of translational research at its institutes and launching the Clinical and Translational Science Award program in 2006.[1-4] Another way of looking at translational research is to see it as research cooperativity between laboratory (bench) and clinic (bedside) scientists (**Figure 4.1**). The translational research process in some ways helps to "connect the dots" between bits of knowledge gleaned from basic research; as more dots are connected, a picture begins to emerge, sufficient for knowledge transfer to the clinical application domain.

Bridging the chasm between basic science and clinical practice is the domain of translational research and one for which evidence-based decision making is well suited. The end point of translational research is properly evaluating an intervention that holds promise—one that can be used clinically or commercialized (brought to market). This process is essential, serving the purpose of translating novel information and mechanisms that have been elucidated through basic science research into practical interventions that can be used in humans to enhance their health.

A foundational objective of translational research is ensuring that the knowledge and beneficial interventions generated by research actually reach the target population. Because the development of a new procedure, intervention, or drug is only the first step, translational research also aims to improve access to people who might benefit from the research. This additional objective requires changes in the infrastructure to eventually

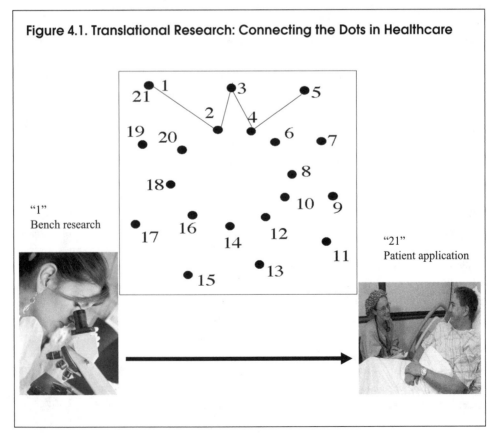

Figure 4.1. Translational Research: Connecting the Dots in Healthcare

"1"
Bench research

"21"
Patient application

have providers and patients engaging in behaviors that encourage research utilization. This ambitious process can be described as 4 phases, each having unique identifying characteristics, yet overlapping greatly with one another (**Table 4.1**).

Table 4.1. The Phases of Translational Research

Phase	Description
1	Seeks to move a basic discovery into a candidate health application.
2	Assesses the value of phase 1 applications for health interventions leading to the development of evidence-based guidelines.
3	Attempts to move evidence-based guidelines into health practice through delivery, dissemination, and utilization of clinical research.
4	Aims to evaluate the "real-world" health outcomes of a phase 1 application once it is incorporated into widespread practice.

The phases described are expected to have considerable overlap, providing feedback loops to permit the integration of new knowledge as it surfaces. Because of the extensive amount of feedback that occurs among the phases, integration of new knowledge is facilitated. The evidence-based practice component of translational research is increasingly revealed as one advances through each of the successive phases.

Translating the knowledge (and lessons) of research into the domain of clinical practice is an extremely complex, multilayer process. As Certified Registered Nurse Anesthetists, we find ourselves at what I term the "sharp end," where the vast domain of knowledge, resources, and interventions interface with and are focused on the target patient (see Figure 2.1). However, many other factors fulfill essential roles in the process of translational research besides the practitioner—these are factors I term "blunt end" factors. A partial list of blunt-end factors includes healthcare policy makers, healthcare insurance companies, funding agencies, pharmaceutical companies, manufacturers of biomedical technology, public health officials, hospital and institutional resources, hospital and institutional governing boards, and the biomedical research community.

In many cases, I believe a sound argument can be constructed that if more resources were directed toward promoting the delivery of existing interventions than in producing new ones, patients might better benefit. Let me give a couple of examples. In the 1840s, the Viennese-based obstetrician Ignaz Philipp Semmelweis introduced mandatory hand washing among his staff, leading to the virtual elimination of childbirth (puerperal) fever, which at the time carried a 20% mortality. Simply washing hands between patients virtually eliminated this catastrophic complication. Yet today, about 10% of the 35 million patients admitted to US hospitals acquire a nosocomial infection, with estimates that many tens of thousands of these patients will die as a result.[5] The cost of treating these infections totals approximately $4.5 to $7.5 billion. Failed hand washing is considered a major cause in this sobering situation.[4-7]

Sometimes (not always) complex problems have simple solutions, the so-called Ockham's razor approach (Sir William of Ockham proposed this principle in the 14th century). What if we engaged in an all-out educational campaign about the essentials of hand washing and rewarded practitioners for engaging in this behavior? What if we put up signage and signal lights as reminders and developed, manufactured, and deployed small, portable, personal hand cleansing devices for every healthcare provider—a little dispenser of liquid or spray that attached to our belt or scrubs or clothing so that it was with us all the time? And to that device we added a little alarm or reminder that every so often cued us to cleanse our hands. Or we installed more sinks in locations proximate to patient care? Or we ensured that hand sanitizer was even more widespread and helped to motivate people to use it? Or we installed ubiquitous, low-cost scanners that emit a specific light wavelength and cause a bright fluorescence when contaminated hands are placed under them? These are simple solutions to a widespread and often catastrophic problem.

Another example comes to mind as well. We are spending a lot of money today developing ever more powerful and ever more expensive antiplatelet drugs. Policy makers, insurance company leaders, healthcare institution administrators, drug company executives, and patients agree that there is a chasm in the access, quality, and disparities in healthcare delivery. Might we narrow the chasm just a bit by doing a better job of having the target populations take their daily low-dose aspirin and monitor its effect?

I do not mean to imply that a simplistic approach is the answer for all healthcare woes. Enlightened people recognize that there is far too much basic science that has not made it to the clinical setting, which in itself tends to demonstrate that a chasm exists. This is a controversy that rages on and is unlikely to reach a reasonable conclusion in the near (or even distant) future.

Example Voyages of Translational Research in Anesthesia Care

Anesthesiology has many examples of long voyages nicely navigated by translational research. Consider just 4 of many translational research domains in anesthesia care: (1) recognition of the importance of nitric oxide, (2) pharmacogenetics, (3) diabetic cardiomyopathy, and (4) perfluorocarbon (PFC)-based oxygen-carrying solutions.

Nitric Oxide as a Nonorganic Physiological Marvel?

Nitric oxide (NO) has had a curious evolution in biomedical research. Not very long ago, this nonorganic molecule was essentially viewed as a pollutant—an environmental menace. Scientists attempting to isolate endothelium-derived relaxant factor were stunned (yet rewarded with the 1998 Nobel Prize for Medicine and Physiology) with their discovery that the simple molecule, NO, was in fact this endogenous vasodilating factor.

Today, as a result of basic research and the harnessing of this knowledge, courtesy of translational research, we know that there are several NO isoforms: neuronal, endothelial, and inducible. The NO molecule is ubiquitous in the body, with a physiological resume as diverse as virtually any other known endogenous substance. Its many essential roles include pain modulation, vascular tone, inflammatory processes, sleep cycling, memory formation, and platelet activity to mention a few. It currently is dispensed to treat erectile dysfunction and dilate the pulmonary vasculature and has been used as a rescue intervention in cases of acute vaso-occlusive crisis resulting from sickle cell disease. The drug is now used in the operating room as part of the anesthesia care of patients, and some modern anesthesia machines are tooled to provide for its administration.

Pharmacogenetics in Anesthesia Comes of Age

Prolonged apnea and paralysis following the administration of succinylcholine, exacerbation of acute porphyria by thiopental, and the perplexing, catastrophic syndrome of malignant hyperthermia were problems that became well recognized in the early 1960s. Contemporary students and practitioners largely take for granted that the foundations of pharmacogenetics and translational research led to our understanding of and development of interventions to manage genetic-based issues related to pseudocholinesterase, aberrant heme synthesis, and the ryanodine receptor in each of these respective issues.

The contemporary recognition of evolutionary biology's relevance to the healthcare of humans would likely have delighted Charles Darwin were he alive today. It was Darwin in his explorations and analyses more than 150 years ago who came to the recognition that the human body can best be understood by the systematic study and appreciation of its evolutionary past. The relevance of evolution to current care strategies is idealized in the modern field of "personalized medicine," in which highly sophisticated approaches are brought to bear on the matter of individualizing care based on genetic analysis. The central thesis to this approach rests firmly on our recognition, achieved via basic science research, that there is enormous individual variation among humans. Darwin incited the effort, one that has hybridized into what we now know as pharmacogenetics. This field is directed at revealing and using to advantage the subtle and not-so-subtle variations that make each of us genetically unique and, thus, often variable in our response to drugs and other interventions. The connectivity between Darwin's voyage on the *HMS Beagle* in 1831 and today's approaches to individualizing a plan of care for a patient based on his or her unique genetic profile seems as real to me as do the connection between the microscope and telescope and advances in bacteriology and astronomy (**Figure 4.2**).

Given advances in pharmacogenetics and the influence of the translational research movement, it is clear that in the near future we will become much better at predicting a patient's response to a given drug, something that has long been a holy grail of clinicians. Enormous advances in molecular biology have enabled us to begin to better identify links between a unique patient's genetic profile and response to a particular drug. Consider the absent analgesia response in some patients who lack the appropriate factor that converts the prodrug codeine to morphine. At its essence, pharmacogenetics is grounded in the complex molecular mechanisms that predict a unique patient's response to drug metabolism, efficacy, and side effects (**Figure 4.3**). This can only further assist us in optimizing individualized decision making predicated on the best evidence when caring for patients in and out of the operating room.

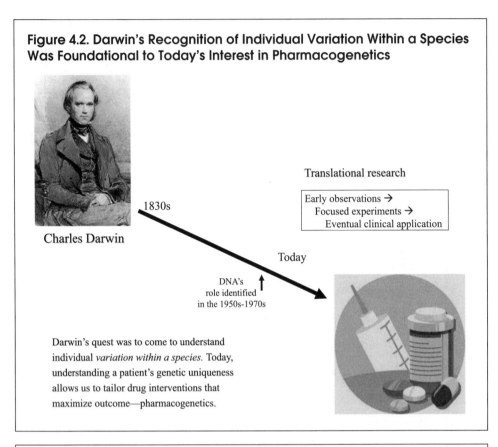

Figure 4.2. Darwin's Recognition of Individual Variation Within a Species Was Foundational to Today's Interest in Pharmacogenetics

Charles Darwin

1830s

Translational research

Early observations →
  Focused experiments →
    Eventual clinical application

Today

DNA's role identified in the 1950s-1970s

Darwin's quest was to come to understand individual *variation within a species*. Today, understanding a patient's genetic uniqueness allows us to tailor drug interventions that maximize outcome—pharmacogenetics.

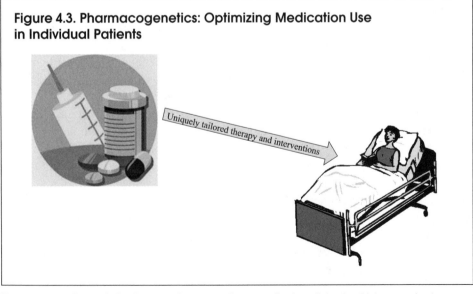

Figure 4.3. Pharmacogenetics: Optimizing Medication Use in Individual Patients

Uniquely tailored therapy and interventions

Pharmacogenetics underlies the current movement, *personalized medicine,* in which recognized individual variations in a patient's genetic makeup allow us to optimize treatment interventions.

Diabetes-Related Heart Failure

Basic science has described the intricacies of the cellular and molecular mechanisms of normal cardiomyocytes, and more recent research is beginning to illuminate the mechanisms of diabetes-induced cardiomyopathy. Diabetes is occurring on a pandemic scale, and its incidence is expected only to increase. Diabetic cardiomyopathy manifests clinically as a decrease in myocardial performance that can occur separate from any related vascular disease. Patients with diabetes undergoing cardiac and noncardiac surgery can be especially challenging to manage because induction of anesthesia is often associated with myocardial depression and hypotension, even in healthy patients without diabetes. However, anesthesia-induced myocardial depression may also have an important role in mediating myocardial protection because anesthetic agents are known to reduce myocardial damage in the setting of ischemia-reperfusion injury. To date, research has not delineated all of the fundamental cellular and molecular mechanisms underlying diabetic cardiomyopathy, and the interactions between anesthetics and proteins involved in regulating myocardial performance and protection are even less well understood. This is an important domain of translational research and one that will likely lead to better understanding and target interventions in this expanding and very challenging patient population.

Perfluorocarbon-Based Oxygen-Carrying Solutions

During the Manhattan Project, begun during World War II, what ultimately emerged was what we now know as nuclear weaponry. Perfluorocarbon chemistry, first studied in the 1930s, was used in that weaponry research to create a protective housing to prevent dangerous corrosion of the inner core of the weapon from the intensely reactive uranium-based material. This research ultimately had a major role in finalizing the bombs that were dropped on Hiroshima, Japan, on August 6, 1945, and on Nagasaki on August 9 of that same year.

Eventually, the Dupont Chemical Company, advancing on the fundamental chemistry of PFCs, developed its product, Teflon. Today many of us find this material in our kitchens and are very familiar with it as a coating to prevent adhesion of food during the cooking process. In the course of this research, it was serendipitously discovered that PFCs were clear, odorless, volatile, nonconducting, and nonflammable and seemed not to be metabolized by the body. But what really caught researchers' attention was that PFCs had an amazing ability to ferry oxygen and carbon dioxide and release both down a concentration gradient. In addition, PFCs proved to be x-ray–opaque so that clinicians could observe their dispersion in the lung.

Further basic research led to PFC emulsification with water, sodium chloride, and egg products (sounds very similar to propofol). The milky white end product has been clinically applied in interventions ranging from partial- and total-liquid ventilation to an intravenous, short-term substitute for blood transfusion. Because a PFC molecule is much smaller than a red blood cell, it is also actively being studied as an intervention when the blood supply is limited because of narrow or obliterated conducting vessels (eg, in head trauma, the vaso-occlusive condition that afflicts people with sickle cell disease, and myocardial infarction) and as an oxygen-carrying solution in conditions of hemorrhage when blood may not be immediately available. The basic science history and the potential patient applications of PFC chemistry represent a storied voyage of translational research.

Final Remarks

Successful health interventions require the translation of a number of other basic sciences besides those that go on at the laboratory bench. These include communication science, psychology, epidemiology, political science, economics, marketing, and others. It is important to recognize that poverty, disparity, language, and culture may play as much of a role as microbiology, physiology, biochemistry, and genetics in marshalling evidence-based care to the bedside. Translational research is an ongoing, enormously complex process of marshaling resources to the task of optimizing healthcare interventions and improving access for the people who need it.

Discovering better ways to ensure that patients receive the care they need—safely, compassionately, and when they need it—poses formidable methodologic challenges. New devices and drugs are fascinating to healthcare providers and the public as well; certainly, they represent major revenue generators for the industries that produce them. However, healthcare decision making must occur with a balance among the need to constantly seek improvement, the goal to maintain reasonable economics, and the mandate to ensure patient advocacy at each stage of the process.

Research targeting the domain of anesthesia care has been aggressively and successfully engaged in by nurse anesthetists, anesthesiologists, pharmacologists, physiologists, and scientists from a wide range of basic science arenas. Given the movement of our profession to the doctoral level (practice doctorate, research doctorate), clinician scientists are being produced in numbers previously never before seen. As such, there is no risk of an intellectual malaise. Nurse anesthetists work in an incredibly patient-centric and data-rich milieu, one in which translational research can readily be used to advantage. When opportunity and need are met by talent and resources, great things can be achieved.

As the sharp-end users of the information, drugs, technologies, and interventions produced by basic and clinical research, anesthesia providers are charged with using the principles of evidence-based decision making in the care we provide. In that process, we must include comparative clinical effectiveness, safety, feasibility, and cost-effectiveness as logical goals in the continuum of translational research. Doing so makes each of us an important player in the translational research continuum and further identifies our role in ensuring that only evidence-based processes associated with quality healthcare delivery actually reach patients.

Figure 4.4 illustrates how translational research should work. It is very much a multidimensional process in which communication must be bidirectional for it to work. Clinical researchers communicate their needs and observations to laboratory researchers to seek the innovations that they need. Members of the public, clinicians in practice, and other professionals in the community communicate their needs and desires for health innovations to researchers. The overall goal is to hasten, and make more efficient, research discoveries that will have more rapid and effective applications to the health needs of society.

Figure 4.4. How Translational Research Should Work!

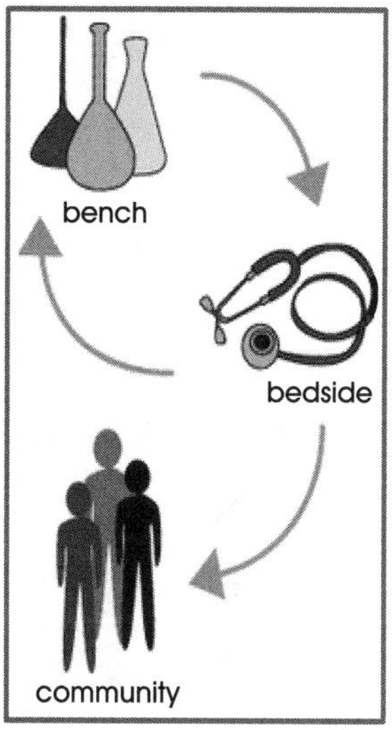

To us knowledge, how good and lovely soever it be for its own sake, must always be a by-end, a step merely towards the still better and lovelier goal of good-will towards men.

Thomas King Chambers, 1850

My interpretation of Chambers and a direct application to the professional world in the 21st century

Everything that we do has ultimately got to be for the goodwill of everyone in our society.

What the National Institutes of Health suggests:

"Translational research includes two areas of translation. One is the process of applying discoveries generated during research in the laboratory, and in preclinical studies, to the development of trials and studies in humans. The second area of translation concerns research aimed at enhancing the adoption of best practices in the community."

(From http://commonfund.nih.gov/clinicalresearch/overview-translational.aspx)

References

1. Travis K. Translational research careers. *Science.* August 17, 2007. http://sciencecareers.sciencemag.org/career_development/previous_issues/articles/2007_08_17/caredit_a0700116/(parent)/68. Accessed September 12, 2012.

2. Fixsen DL, Naoom SF, Blase KA, Friedman RM, Wallace F. *Implementation Research: A Synthesis of the Literature.* Tampa, FL: National Implementation Research Network, Louis de la Parte Florida Mental Health Institute (FMHI), University of South Florida; 2005. FMHI publication No. 231. http://nirn.fpg.unc.edu/resources/implementation-research-synthesis-literature. Accessed September 12, 2012.

3. Agency for Healthcare Research and Quality. Translating Research Into Practice II (TRIP II) information conference: summary. Rockville, MD: Agency for Healthcare Research and Quality; February 2, 2000. http://www.ahrq.gov/fund/tripconf.htm#head2. Accessed September 12, 2012.

4. Fontanarosa PB, DeAngelis CD. Basic science and translational research in *JAMA* [editorial]. *JAMA.* 2002;287(13):1728.

5. Klevens RM, Edwards JR, Richards CL Jr, et al. Estimating health care-associated infections and death in U.S. hospitals. *Public Health Rep.* 2007;122(2):160-166.

6. Wenzel RP, Edmond MB. The impact of hospital-acquired bloodstream infections. *Emerg Infect Dis.* 2001;7(2):174-177.

7. Centers for Disease Control and Prevention. Handwashing: clean hands save lives. http://www.cdc.gov/handwashing. Accessed September 12, 2012.

CHAPTER FIVE

Is the Almighty P Becoming Less So? Reconsidering the Significance of "Statistical Significance"

As a matter of tradition, there is great reliance in the biomedical literature on the use of P values to test and confer importance to hypotheses. This reliance continues to be commonplace. To further illustrate its deep roots in professional cultures, it is not uncommon to hear clinicians and researchers alike exclaim that "a P value less than .001 is more significant than a P value less than .05" in attesting to some finding from a study. But what does such reporting of a P value do for us, or, more to the point, what is P?

The P Value Deconstructed

P values represent nothing more than a metric of the strength of the evidence for or against the *null hypothesis*. For example, a study is performed looking at the speed of emergence (perhaps defined as "the patient follows the command to squeeze one's hand") in pediatric patients undergoing tonsillectomy who are randomized to a propofol–nitrous oxide–opiate–based anesthetic compared with a sevoflurane–nitrous oxide–opiate–based anesthetic. The null hypothesis is that there is no difference between the groups in the selected emergence outcome. Rejection of the null hypothesis suggests that there is a difference in the measured outcome that could be related to the intervention that was applied (ie, propofol or sevoflurane). The P value ascribes a degree of evidence that the observed difference is due to the manipulation that was performed rather than simply chance. It is not a measure of the magnitude of the effect. Thus, we frequently hear of concerns related to "statistical vs clinical significance" of a study's findings or conclusions.

A study that reports a low P value (eg, $P = .024$) suggests that there is little risk that chance alone accounted for any observed differences, instead urging consideration that the experimental manipulation was responsible. A high P value (eg, $P > .083$) urges consideration of the groups as equivalent in their response to the manipulations and acceptance of the null hypothesis (ie, no effect/no difference). As stated, traditionally, a P value less than .05 has been most often identified as the demarcation between "significant" and "not significant." Precisely why a chance effect of less than 1 in 20 ($P < .05$) represents significance is historically unclear but appears inextricably embedded in our culture. The P metric is a kind of icon that lives on as a de facto "almighty" value.

Importance of Effect Size Measures

Effect size measures are increasingly encountered as a way that helps to put into perspective the magnitude of the effect of a manipulation, whether the outcome of interest is the duration of a drug course, rating of an intervention's efficacy, core temperature, pain score, cost of an intervention, laboratory value, or any of a multitude of other assessments of clinical interest. Effect size quantifies the magnitude of an intervention compared with another, rather than simply a form of black or white, yes or no, dichotomous categorization of significant or not significant. For clinicians, this movement provides a real-world characterization of the degree of impact that a particular intervention has relative to one or more other interventions.

The *Publication Manual of the American Psychological Association* indicates that in reporting a research finding, "it is almost always necessary to include some index of effect size or strength of relationship."[1] This was advocated more than a decade earlier by Cohen,[2] the statistical power guru, who wrote that "the primary product of a research inquiry is one of measures of effect size, not P values." There has been a gradual, if not lethargic, national movement in this direction. Indeed, some journal editors now require authors to report effect size measures. The *AANA Journal* encourages the reporting of such measures but, for a variety of reasons, including a lack of grassroots appreciation and the traditional conservativeness of research reporting traditions, has not made the inclusion mandatory.

Effect size measures provide essential information that is much different from simply reporting the α level (P value). Effect size addresses the clinical and practical importance of the results of a research finding. Frequently, a statistically significant result is reported that does not have practical (clinical) significance. One basic misunderstanding in statistical analysis is thinking that an observed P value that is considered highly significant, for example P = .0001, also reflects a large effect. The P value simply represents the likelihood that an observed finding is due to chance or sampling error and reveals nothing about the size of the effect. In the most elemental description, the P value is useful in indicating if there is the presence or absence of an effect, whereas the effect size quantifies the degree of the observed effect. One important reason to use effect size measures is that they can help researchers consider the clinical or practical importance of the findings apart from mere statistical significance.

Examples of Effect Size Measures

A *confidence interval* is the range in which something is anticipated to occur. Of course, the prediction (anticipation) might be incorrect; the degree of confidence measures the probability of that expectation to be true.

Frequently, a "95% confidence interval" is reported. The degree of confidence is wedded to the width of the confidence interval. One can be fairly confident that something will be within a very broad range and less confident with a very narrow range. The sample size that the observation has been drawn from greatly influences the width of the confidence interval. The more information accumulated in making observations of a phenomenon, the greater the confidence that the measure or observation will be within the selected interval. As a corollary, as more information is accumulated and as confidence increases, the interval narrows. A 95% confidence interval implies that 19 of 20 times, the true value will be in the specified range.

The *odds ratio* and the *relative risk* assess the likelihood of an event between 2 comparison groups. Consider the following fictional data set of all-cause mortality of middle-aged smokers and nonsmokers living in a rural locale. In the modestly sized sample are 462 nonsmokers and 851 smokers. The epidemiologic study tracked these 2 cohorts (a *cohort* is simply a well-defined group) for 15 years, and, at the end of that time, the findings were reported. The follow-up reveals that 308 nonsmokers were alive and 154 had died. With respect to the 851 smokers, 142 were alive and 709 had died (**Table 5.1**).

Table 5.1. Outcome for Smokers vs Nonsmokers in a 15-Year Study

	Alive	Dead	Total
Nonsmokers	308	154	462
Smokers	142	709	851
Total	450	863	1,313

The data in the table make it pretty obvious that smokers were more likely to have died during the study period than were nonsmokers. Although it is clear that statistical significance would be demonstrable, the fundamental question is "How much more likely is a smoker to die than a nonsmoker?" Traditional statistical testing does not answer this question but reveals only whether there is a statistically significant difference between the cohorts in their rate of death at the 15-year follow-up. The odds ratio and the relative risk can be used to shed light on this question.

Humans are generally quite comfortable in considering the odds of something happening. Consider the example of rolling a die. The odds of rolling a 6 on a fair die are 5:1 against getting a 6. The odds ratio compares the predicted odds of an event occurring when some factor is or is not present.

In the current example, the odds ratio compares the relative odds of death in each group. For nonsmokers, the odds are 2 to 1 against dying (154/308 = 0.5). For smokers, the odds are nearly 5 to 1 in favor of death (709/142 = 4.993). The odds ratio is computed (4.993/0.5 = 9.99), demonstrating an almost 10-fold greater odds of death for smokers compared with nonsmokers in the fictional sampled population.

The relative risk (sometimes called the *risk ratio*) compares the probability of death in the comparison groups rather than the odds. For nonsmokers, the probability of death during the study period is 33% (ie, No. of Deaths/Total No. of Nonsmokers, or 154/462 = 0.3333). For smokers on the other hand, the probability is 83% (709/851 = 0.8331). The relative risk of death is 2.5 (0.8331/0.3333 = 2.5). The conclusion is that there is a 2.5 greater probability of death for smokers than for nonsmokers.

The magnitude of these measures is quite different in this example. Although both reveal that smokers were more likely to die during the study period, which of the measures is a more accurate representation of reality? This is not always an easy question to answer but an important one to consider as one weighs the evidence. A number of issues are operative, but, in general, relative risk measures events in a way that is generally consistent with our thinking, that is, if the risk is 1, the exposure is not associated with the outcome. With an increased risk, the ratio is greater than 1; if there is decreased risk, the ratio is less than 1. *Relative risk* is a relative measure and is the ratio of the risk in the exposed group to that in the unexposed group. The *odds ratio* is the ratio of the odds of having the event in the exposed group to that in the unexposed group. These 2 measures are suitable for different purposes and appeal to different people in different ways. For a variety of computational reasons, the odds ratio is better suited for use in logistic regression (Chapter 12) and case-control studies. In addition, the odds ratio is better suited when the outcome of interest is relatively rare because it tends to overestimate risk in a manner similar to the preceding nonsmoker vs smoker example (**Figure 5.1**).

Application to the Framingham Heart Study

In 1948, the Framingham Heart Study, under the direction of the National Heart, Lung, and Blood Institute, began an ambitious project in health research. The investigators recruited 5,209 healthy men and women between the ages of 30 and 62 years from the town of Framingham, Massachusetts. The researchers performed extensive physical examinations and lifestyle inventories; the surviving subjects have continued to return to the study every 2 years for a detailed medical history, physical examination, and laboratory tests. The initial and primary goal of the study was to identify common factors and individual characteristics that contributed to the development of cardiovascular disorders. The results of the ongoing study have been published over the years with relative risk and odds ratios used to quantify many of the research findings.

In a now classic finding from the Framingham Heart Study that used an effect size measure, the investigators examined the mortality of subjects 55 to 94 years of age in whom atrial fibrillation (AF) developed during 40 years of follow-up of the original participants.[3] Of the original 5,209 subjects, AF developed in 296 men and 325 women (mean ages, 74 and 76 years, respectively). The investigators used pooled logistic regression, and after they adjusted for age, hypertension, smoking, diabetes, left ventricular hypertrophy, myocardial infarction, congestive heart failure, valvular heart disease, and stroke or transient ischemic attack, AF was associated with an odds ratio for death of 1.5 (95% confidence interval, 1.2 to 1.8) in men and 1.9 (95% confidence interval, 1.5 to 2.2) in women. In the Framingham Heart Study, AF remained significantly associated with excess mortality, with about a doubling of mortality in both sexes.

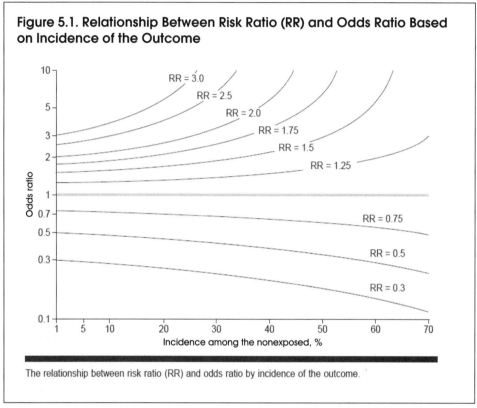

Figure 5.1. Relationship Between Risk Ratio (RR) and Odds Ratio Based on Incidence of the Outcome

The relationship between risk ratio (RR) and odds ratio by incidence of the outcome.

The odds ratio and risk ratio are both commonly referred to as "relative risk" metrics. Although in many conditions they can be used without too much inherent pitfall, only under certain conditions do they truly approximate one another. The figure reveals that when the outcome of interest becomes more frequent, the odds ratio will overestimate the risk ratio when it is > 1 and will tend to underestimate the risk ratio when it is < 1.

The authors concluded that in the studied subjects, AF was associated with a 1.5- to 1.9-fold mortality risk after adjustment for the preexisting cardiovascular conditions with which AF was related. The decreased survival seen with AF was present in men and women across a wide range of ages.

Other Common Effect Size Measures

The *number needed to treat* (NNT) indicates the number of patients required to be treated to avoid 1 adverse outcome event, such as postoperative vomiting after gynecologic surgery or thromboembolism following joint arthroplasty. For example, if a drug has an NNT of 8, it implies that 8 people must be treated with the drug to prevent 1 additional bad outcome. A drug or an intervention with a low NNT would be considered to have a greater magnitude of effect than a comparable drug or intervention with a high NNT. The NNT is frequently used in reporting findings from a large randomized controlled trial

(Chapter 3) or in reporting a pooled estimate based on a number of high-quality trials such as in a meta-analysis (Chapter 7). Given the importance of the NNT metric and its increasingly common use in the anesthesia literature, Chapter 6 focuses on understanding the strengths and limitations of the NNT.

The *Pearson r correlation* is a widely used effect size measure. It can be used when the data are continuous or binary; thus, the Pearson *r* may be the most versatile of the effect size measures currently available. This was the first important effect size metric to be developed in statistics. The Pearson *r* can vary in magnitude from −1.0 to +1.0, with −1.0 indicating a perfect negative linear relation, +1.0 indicating a perfect positive linear relation, and 0 indicating no relation between 2 variables. Although interpretations tend to vary somewhat, a useful if not somewhat arbitrary guideline is that values between 0.2 and 0.4 represent a mild association between variables; values between 0.5 and 0.7, a moderate association; and values of 0.8 to 1.0, a strong association. (See Figure 12.2 for a discussion of correlation.)

A further mathematical manipulation of the correlation coefficient is to square the value (r^2), which represents the *coefficient of determination*. This calculation is used to represent an estimation of how much a change in one variable influences the other.

The *Cohen d* is an effect size measure to use in the context of a *t* test that compares group means. Formulaically, *d* is defined as the difference between 2 means divided by the standard deviation (SD) for those means. In developing this tool, Cohen proposed that the SD of either group could be used when the variances of the 2 groups were similar. The interpretation of *d* is as follows: 0.2 denotes a small effect; 0.5, a medium effect; and 0.8, a large effect size. One drawback of using the Cohen *d* is that the outcome is strongly influenced by the denominator of the equation. If one SD is larger than the other, the denominator is weighted in that direction and the effect size is tilted toward a more conservative measure.

Yet another effect size measure is the *Hedges g,* named for one of the early champions of meta-analysis, Gene Glass. It incorporates sample size by computing a denominator that looks at the sample sizes of the respective SDs and adjusts the overall effect size on the basis of this sample size.

The *Cohen f^2* is the appropriate effect size measure to use in the context of an F test for multiple correlation or multiple regression. By convention, f^2 effect sizes of 0.02, 0.15, and 0.35 are considered small, medium, and large, respectively. The *Cramer Phi* (ϕ) is yet another effect size measure, and it is a good measure of association for the χ^2 test.

Statistical Power: What Is a Power Analysis and What Are Type I and II Errors?

It would be premature to end this discussion without considering the issue of *statistical power*. Earlier, the notion of hypothesis testing was introduced, suggesting that traditional statistical analysis informs whether to accept or reject the null hypothesis. Incorrectly rejecting the null hypothesis—concluding that a difference between or among the groups exists when, in fact, one does not—constitutes what is known as a *type I (α) error*. When a difference exists between or among the groups and is not detected, the null hypothesis has been falsely accepted, which is a *type II (β) error* (**Table 5.2**). How can these 2 types of common errors in hypothesis testing be minimized?

Table 5.2. Type I and Type II Errors

What the research revealed	The real-world situation	
	The null hypothesis is actually TRUE.	The alternative hypothesis is actually TRUE.
The null hypothesis is found to be TRUE.	😊 Correct	🙁 Incorrect, type II error
The alternative hypothesis is found to be TRUE.	🙁 Incorrect, type I error	😊 Correct

Type I error claims an effect (a difference) that does not exist.
Type II error claims no effect (or no difference) when one exists.

The concept of *power* relates to the ability of the test to detect an interventional effect if such an effect is truly present; researchers deal with this by doing a *power analysis*. A number of factors are considered in planning and performing a power analysis, including the following:

- The level set for the risk of making a type I error (ie, the α or P value). This level is often (not always) set at .05.
- The level set to detect an effect that represents β, the risk of a type II error, and the power being $1 - \beta$. This level is often (but not always) set at .80.
- The effect size, an estimation of the magnitude of the trend or relationship that exists between the independent and dependent variables
- The anticipated variation in the measured response based on previous research
- The type of statistical tool that will be used
- The sample size (N)

For example, to determine if one form of convective warming device is different from another in efficacy, a clinical trial is designed and attempts to control for as many confounding variables as possible (eg, patient randomization, surgery duration, intravenous fluid amount, type of anesthetic, and room temperature). A question posed before the start of the study is "What is the size of a clinically important difference that we want to detect?" The researchers want to quantify the distance between the null hypothesis (no group differences) and a preidentified value that represents the alternative hypothesis (one group more or less than the other) that is of clinical or practical value.

Effect sizes are classified by their magnitude. Given our understanding of a relationship present between or among the variables under study and our threshold for detecting a meaningful difference, an established formula can be used for actually computing the number of subjects needed in each of the convective warming groups to accomplish the task. The concept of power is a bit like making sure that the fuel in a car has sufficient octane to do its job.

A study that is underpowered will likely fail to detect an effect that is actually present or may simply provide indecisive results. However, a study can be overpowered as well. Researchers may demonstrate that an effect is present, even though the actual difference may be trivial and below the level of practical or clinical relevance.

For a definitive discussion of power and its theoretical foundation, readers are referred to Cohen's seminal text, *Statistical Power Analysis for the Behavioral Sciences.*[2] Cohen's text contains formulas for researchers who need to do these calculations. In addition, formulas are available on the Internet by simply searching for "statistical power calculation formula."

Final Thoughts

Effect size measures are increasingly being used (and sometimes required) in research reports and represent a substantial improvement over conventional hypothesis testing in conveying the findings of research. Effect size reporting provides a metric of the magnitude of effect of an intervention, yet, despite the advantages of effect size measures over the reporting of *P* values alone, many of us remain largely unaware of their value. Further discussion and a table of common effect size measures can be found in Chapter 7 (on meta-analysis).

References

1. American Psychological Association. *Publication Manual of the American Psychological Association.* 5th ed. Washington, DC: American Psychological Association; 2001:25.

2. Cohen J. *Statistical Power Analysis for the Behavioral Sciences.* Hillsdale, NJ: Lawrence Erlbaum Associates; 1988:12.

3. Benjamin E, Wolf P, D'Agostino R, Silbershatz H, Kannel W, Levy D. Impact of atrial fibrillation on the risk of death: the Framingham Heart Study. *Circulation.* 1998;98(10):946-952.

CHAPTER SIX

Understanding the Strengths and Limitations of the "Number Needed to Treat"

Mentioned in Chapter 5, and deserving of further consideration here, the *number needed to treat* (NNT) is an extremely common metric seen in research reports and systematic reviews that helps us better understand the evidence relative to an intervention. The following poem beautifully captures the essence of the measure and its application in our evidence-based decision making:

"Number Needed To Treat

It rolls off the tongue
  six syllables
    four words
      two parts with a taste
of alliteration.

A number derived
  from faith in numbers
    and the sacrifice of number one
      upon the altar
of absolute risk reduction.

It teaches
  treating one patient
    is rarely enough
      to make a difference
to one patient.

It promises
  cast this pill
    into this many stomachs
      and one day in at least one patient
your wish will come true.

One after another my patients thank me
  for something
    that will probably do nothing
      except for that one—
eeny meeny miny moe."

(Reprinted with kind permission of the author, Adam Possner, MD. © 2011, *Journal of the American Medical Association.*)

As argued earlier in this book, there is an increasing awakening among researchers and clinicians (as well as journal editors) that one cannot ignore the magnitude of an effect and simply focus on the statistical significance of an intervention. The confidence interval is one approach to this issue in that it provides information not only about the size of the effect but also the statistical relationship. Yet even this metric may fall short of the mark and in many situations an even more robust and meaningful metric of the magnitude of effect is desired. Highly amenable to this is the NNT.

The NNT provides a robust look at the absolute change in risk associated with an intervention. The NNT is the average number of patients that we would expect to "treat" (ie, perform an intervention on) in order to achieve 1 observed, desired outcome. An NNT that is low (eg, NNT = 2 or 3) suggests that we would see the expected outcome frequently in patients whom we treat, whereas with an NNT of 200 or 300, we would need to apply the intervention to a large number of patients to see an effect.

Recently I read a new book, intended for the lay public, about how they should become active participants in their medical decision making.[1] Although humans generally consider themselves rational in their decision making, choices made with respect to healthcare are complex and associated with many unknowns. One example the authors use is dealing with prostate cancer, a slowly progressing process, such that more men die with it than of it. The authors cite compelling research noting that if 48 prostate surgeries are performed, only 1 patient benefits from it, yet many are harmed by it (infection, bleeding, incontinence, impotence, etc). There is strong evidence that the likelihood of at least one of these side effects occurring is about 50%, that is, 24 of the 47 who do not benefit from the surgery will have an adverse consequence. The decision to have or not have the surgery is complex at best.

Consider yet another hypothetical example discussed by the authors (one is a Harvard oncologist; the other, a Harvard endocrinologist). A newly released drug is found to reduce the risk of a catastrophic illness by 50%, yet the incidence of the illness overall is about 1 in 1,000. If you take the drug and experience a 50% reduction in experiencing the illness, you now have a 1 in 2,000 chance of contracting the illness. Although this may be a good thing, it would be important to know what adverse consequences are associated with the therapy. Better understanding the likelihood of adversity with the therapy can be illuminated by what is known as the *number needed to harm* (NNH), which is discussed in the next section.

For those readers who are mathematically inclined, the calculation for the NNT looks like this:

$$NNT = 1.0 / (P1 - P2)$$

where P1 is the proportion of the outcome interest in the control group and P2 is the proportion of the outcome of interest in the treatment group. When using the NNT, you must have a distinct event, such as "death" or "pain relief achieved" or "hemoglobin of 11 g/dL attained" or "episodes of vomiting." Dealing with continuous data, such as "duration of hypoxemia" or "duration of pain relief" can be amenable to the NNT but would have to be transformed in some way such as "those who have experienced satisfactory oxygenation achieved after 2 hours of therapy" or "the proportion of patients who achieved pain relief in 8 hours" or something along this line.

Let's look at a couple of examples of NNT, the first from the cardiovascular medicine literature and another from the anesthesia literature.

Statin therapy is used in the medical management of cardiovascular risk factors. The Justification for the Use of Statin in Prevention: An Intervention Trial Evaluating Rosuvastatin (JUPITER) study randomized rosuvastatin, 20 mg, or placebo in 17,802 apparently healthy men and women based on their medical history, normal low-density lipoprotein cholesterol, and other factors.[2] Examining **Table 6.1** from the article[2] with respect to the NNT values, we must consider not only the timeframe (eg, 1-year vs 2-year) but also the particular outcome (end point) of interest. The table presents incidence rates and the observed risk reduction associated with the statin, rosuvastatin, compared with placebo over time with respect to the outcomes of myocardial infarction, stroke, hospitalization for unstable angina, revascularization and death. If we look at the 1-year epoch, we see that the NNT was 215 and the 5-year NNT was 25 for the composite primary end point, suggesting an impressive clinical effect over time, not surprising given the relatively low-risk population at the start of the study, the normal evolution of cardiovascular disease, and the known mechanism of action of statin therapy. Although we may wonder why the statin was compared with placebo rather than with another studied intervention, the authors reported that

Table 6.1. Number Needed to Treat (NNT) in Rosuvastatin Trial

	Primary end point	Primary end point[a], or any death	Primary end point, VTE, or any death	Primary revascularization or any death	MI, stroke, or any death
Events, placebo	251	441	483	431	353
Events, rosuvastatin	142	295	320	291	239
Incidence rate[b], placebo	1.36	2.39	2.62	2.23	1.90
Incidence rate[b], rosuvastatin	0.77	1.59	1.73	1.57	1.28
Incidence rate difference	0.59	0.80	0.89	0.76	0.62
Relative risk reduction, %	44	33	34	33	32
1-year NNT	215	158	147	167	164
2-year NNT	95	73	65	76	95
3-year NNT	49	38	33	40	54
4-year NNT	31	25	23	25	36
5-year NNT	25	20	18	20	29

Abbreviations: NNT, number needed to treat; MI, myocardial infarction; VTE, venous thromboembolism.
[a] Primary trial end point is myocardial infarction, stroke, hospitalization for unstable angina, arterial revascularization, or cardiovascular death.
[b] Incidence rate per 100 person-years

the observed preventive value of rosuvastatin is noted to have substantially better NNT values than those associated with antihypertensive or aspirin therapy.

Another example follows from the anesthesia literature. Here the use of ondansetron in the management of postoperative nausea and vomiting (PONV) in children undergoing strabismus repair was examined.[3] The intent was to evaluate the use of prophylactic ondansetron compared with rescue ondansetron treatment in the management of PONV. The NNT to prevent PONV was 2 and the NNT to treat PONV was 9. Although both approaches demonstrated good effectiveness, the prevention strategy ruled! That many of us use ondansetron as a prophylactic antiemetic is based on sound research and has a powerful NNT that informs that practice.

A look at the website Bandolier revealed some interesting NNT values for different medical therapies, as noted below.[4]

- Prevention of postoperative vomiting using droperidol (NNT = 4.4)
- Prevention of infection from dog bites using an antibiotic (NNT = 16)
- Prevention of stroke using a daily, low-dose aspirin for a year (NNT = 102)

Wonder what the NNT is for oseltamivir (Tamiflu) in preventing 1 death from the flu? Recent research demonstrates that it is on the order of 1,800 to 3,200 depending on the assumptions, patient age, and such issues as whether one is looking at all-cause mortality or more stringent influenza-related mortality.[5] Whereas this does not imply that oseltamivir is ineffective (it is quite effective at reducing illness duration and the potential of an infected individual to transmit the condition to another), it provides insight into its limitation if mortality is the sole consideration.

Figure 6.1 illustrates a hypothetical trial of antiemetic therapy. The calculations reveal an NNT of 5 for the new therapy, suggesting a relatively impressive effect.

Number Needed to Harm

The NNH is somewhat analogous to the NNT and is a metric that helps us understand the likelihood of some defined adverse event. It is the number of patients who would need to receive an intervention to cause 1 complication or adverse event associated with that intervention.

A 2003 study looking at laryngeal complications associated with tracheal intubation set out to determine whether the quality of tracheal intubation, based on the use of a nondepolarizer or no relaxant at all, affects the incidence of vocal cord sequelae.[6] The authors concluded that adding a nondepolarizer (compared with none) to a propofol-fentanyl induction sequence was associated with greatly improved quality of tracheal intubation and a markedly decreased rate of postoperative hoarseness and vocal cord complications. The study was properly powered and an NNH of 3.5 for postoperative hoarseness and an NNH of 2.9 for vocal cord sequelae were determined if the nondepolarizer was omitted, suggesting a high rate of adverse consequences when a relaxant is not employed. Although these findings may seem unsurprising to the experienced practitioner, this was, to my

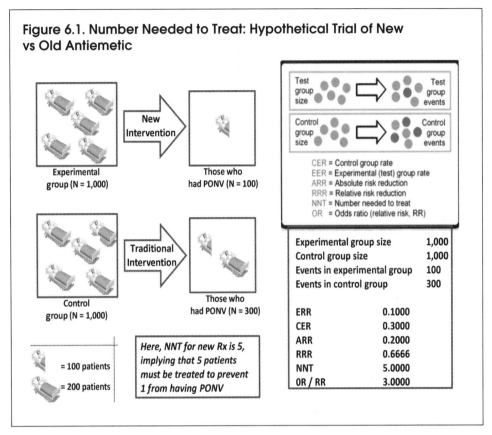

Figure 6.1. Number Needed to Treat: Hypothetical Trial of New vs Old Antiemetic

Abbreviations: PONV, postoperative nausea and vomiting; Rx, prescription.

knowledge, the first study to examine the influence of intubating conditions and induction technique on postoperative hoarseness and vocal cord sequelae.

Final Thoughts and Cautions

Although an NNT and NNH may be reported in a study or review, it should be kept in mind that these values may not be directly applicable to a particular patient. Evidence-based decision making is contextually sensitive (as noted throughout this text) and because of differences in baseline risk, patient characteristics, and even perturbations in the manner in which an intervention is applied by the practitioner, NNT and NNH must be interpreted with care.

When considering the clinical applicability of research findings, carefully scrutinize the reports of trials or systematic reviews for treatment effects based on subgroup analysis. Those that immediately come to mind are subanalyses that look at race, gender, age, comorbidity, and concomitant drug therapy. Even avid proponents of magnitude of effect measures (such as the NNT and NNH) voice concern that when the results of a trial with one baseline risk are applied to a particular patient with different attributes (risk factors), substantially flawed translation can occur[7] (**Figure 6.2**).

The NNT and NNH are merely point estimates and thus are associated with their own predictive liabilities even in the best of circumstances. Confidence intervals are usually employed to indicate the upper and lower limits of the NNT or NNH such that, by convention, we can assume a 95% probability that the real value is in the range reported.

Although the NNT and NNH are relatively easy calculations to perform when dealing with a single trial, things get complicated when data are pooled from multiple trials, as may be the case in a systematic analysis (eg, meta-analysis). Subject variation, as noted above, can be a major issue, and failure to adjust for an individual's baseline characteristics can lead to specious or even dangerous interventions.

Remember that with every NNT report, there is an associated NNH and knowledge of the latter value is vital in deciding the merit of any intervention under consideration. Whereas NNT calculations obtained from a meta-analysis of randomized controlled trials usually provide the best evidence for the intervention's effectiveness, always consider the context sensitivity of that information relative to a particular patient.

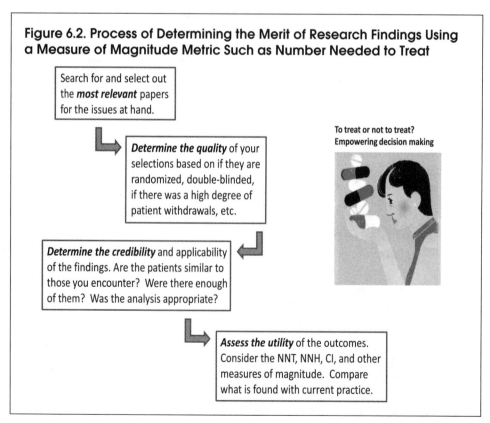

Figure 6.2. Process of Determining the Merit of Research Findings Using a Measure of Magnitude Metric Such as Number Needed to Treat

Search for and select out the ***most relevant*** papers for the issues at hand.

Determine the quality of your selections based on if they are randomized, double-blinded, if there was a high degree of patient withdrawals, etc.

Determine the credibility and applicability of the findings. Are the patients similar to those you encounter? Were there enough of them? Was the analysis appropriate?

Assess the utility of the outcomes. Consider the NNT, NNH, CI, and other measures of magnitude. Compare what is found with current practice.

To treat or not to treat? Empowering decision making

Abbreviations: NNT, number needed to treat; NNH, number needed to harm.

References

1. Groopman J, Hartzband P. *Your Medical Mind: How to Decide What is Right for You.* New York, NY: Penguin Press; 2011.

2. Ridker PM, MacFadyen JG, Francisco AH, et al; JUPITER Study Group. Number needed to treat with rosuvastatin to prevent first cardiovascular events and death among men and women with low low-density lipoprotein cholesterol and elevated high-sensitivity C-reactive protein: justification for the use of statins in prevention: an intervention trial evaluating rosuvastatin (JUPITER). *Circ Cardiovasc Qual Outcomes.* 2009;2(6):616-623.

3. Sennaraj B, Shende D, Sadhasivam S, Ilavajady S, Jagan D. Management of post-strabismus nausea and vomiting in children using odansetron: a value-based comparison of outcomes. *Br J Anaesth.* 2009;89(3):473-478.

4. Bandolier, Website. http://www.medicine.ox.ac.uk/bandolier/. Accessed September 15, 2012.

5. Thompson WW, Shay DK, Weintraub E, et al. Mortality associated with influenza and respiratory syncytial virus in the United States. *JAMA.* 2003;289(2):179-186.

6. Mencke T, Echternach M, Kleinschmidt S, et al. Laryngeal morbidity and quality of tracheal intubation: a randomized controlled trial. *Anesthesiology.* 2003;98(5):1049-1056.

7. Cook RJ, Sackett DL. The number needed to treat: a clinically useful measure of treatment effect [published correction appears in *BMJ.* 1995;310(6986):1056]. *BMJ.* 1995;310(6977):452-454.

CHAPTER SEVEN

A Primer on the Meta-analysis: Precisely Estimating an Intervention's Effect

The *meta-analysis* assumes a prominent place in evidence-based practice search strategies and merits special consideration so that its characteristics and usefulness are best understood. It sits atop the "hierarchy of evidence" (see Figure 2.5) and assists in addressing the question, "Does intervention X offer significant benefit when used in a particular patient group?" when a range of findings is presented in various journals in a number of years for a diverse set of clinical settings.

The *systematic review* (SR) is an explicitly described method by which evidence from the literature involving specific interventions and well-defined outcomes is retrieved in a highly systematic manner. The SRs that are of particularly high quality endeavor to retrieve all relevant and meritorious studies, assess the individual studies for quality, and synthesize the finding from the studies in an unbiased way such that an impartial summary results.

In its most elemental form, the meta-analysis is a quantitative SR. Its purpose is to provide an estimate of the overall benefit (or risk) of an intervention that has been gleaned from carefully selected, randomized controlled trials (RCTs) (**Figure 7.1**). The meta-analysis draws on a heterogeneous group of patients who were studied in a range of trials. Therefore, the meta-analysis achieves increased power to detect any clinically significant effects and proves exacting estimates of the size of any effects that are revealed.

The SR and meta-analysis have become more commonplace in the anesthesia-related literature. Examples include the following:

- Comparing desflurane and isoflurane or propofol with respect to the ability of patients to follow commands on agent discontinuation[1]
- Describing the relative advantages and disadvantages of the laryngeal mask airway compared with face mask or endotracheal tube airway management during general anesthesia[2]
- Elucidating the risk of spontaneous abortion in women whose occupations involve exposure to nitrous oxide[3]
- Defining the relative efficacy and adverse events associated with intrathecal morphine, fentanyl, and sufentanil for postcesarean delivery pain[4]

Figure 7.1. The Meta-analysis

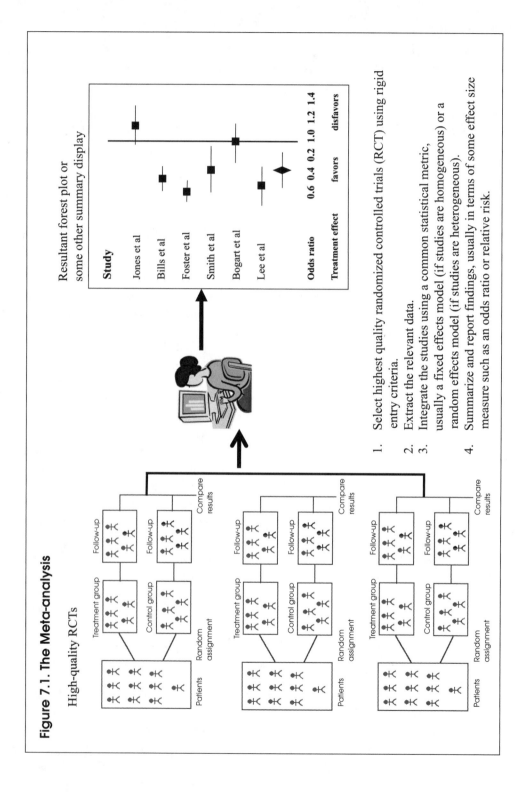

High-quality RCTs

Resultant forest plot or some other summary display

Study	
Jones et al	
Bills et al	
Foster et al	
Smith et al	
Bogart et al	
Lee et al	

Odds ratio   0.6 0.4 0.2 1.0 1.2 1.4

Treatment effect   favors   disfavors

1. Select highest quality randomized controlled trials (RCT) using rigid entry criteria.
2. Extract the relevant data.
3. Integrate the studies using a common statistical metric, usually a fixed effects model (if studies are homogeneous) or a random effects model (if studies are heterogeneous).
4. Summarize and report findings, usually in terms of some effect size measure such as an odds ratio or relative risk.

- Determining the efficacy of epidural analgesia compared with parenteral opioids for postoperative pain relief for a wide range of surgical procedures[5]
- Examining comparative cost, morbidity, and mortality associated with off-pump and conventional coronary artery bypass procedures[6]
- Evaluating the incidence of emergence phenomena in children who are anesthetized with halothane or sevoflurane[7]

In 2002, I reported a meta-analysis that evaluated the effectiveness of nonsteroidal anti-inflammatory agents vs codeine in a standardized pain model.[8] Since that initial effort, I employed similar methods to interrogate a current controversial topic ("To press or not to press, and if so, with what? A single question focused meta-analysis of vasopressor choice during regional anesthesia in obstetrics." *AANA Journal,* August 2013.) These are the only meta-analyses that I could find in the nurse anesthesia literature as of late 2012. To illustrate, the initial search resulted in finding more than 300 studies, of which only 8 were subjected to meta-analysis based on stringent inclusion criteria (eg, RCT with double blinding, appropriately powered, minimum of 2 treatment arms, standardized and valid outcome tools, and consistent follow-up with reporting of adverse events). The results of these studies were transformed into a common metric using established procedures, and the data were analyzed using a technique called the random effects model. The study concluded that overall, nonsteroidal anti-inflammatory agents were as effective as or more effective than codeine and were associated with fewer adverse effects than codeine therapy.

Search for a Common Metric

Different studies, even when pursuing a similar research objective, are unlikely to use the same manner of outcome measurement. Therefore, use of some measure of the effect size (ie, determining the magnitude of effect of the intervention) is most often sought as a common statistical metric in the meta-analysis.

Consider a meta-analysis for which the objective relates to the study of postoperative pain management. A variety of well-performed RCTs are selected from the literature that meet the predetermined inclusion criteria of the SR. The various researchers in the selected studies are likely to have operationalized and, thus, measured postoperative pain in a manner that differs among the pooled studies. For example, different visual analog scales may have been used, some studies may have reported the total mass of drug used, and still others may have selected some other surrogate measure of discomfort. Each of these outcome measures would obviously have varied numerics, means, and standard deviations, so that any attempt at averaging the study results would prove as impossible as averaging gallons, miles, and horsepower in the same equation. The task of the meta-analysis is to translate each of the included studies into a common statistical metric in such a way that the various outcomes that were measured have a similar meaning and, therefore, can be averaged in a meaningful manner.

Brief Overview of the Conduct of the Meta-analysis

Step 1: The Problem or Hypothesis Statement

As with any research study that involves a clinical intervention and an outcome (eg, ultrasound vs electrical stimulation and complications of interscalene block, respectively), performing a meta-analysis demands a focused, clearly written hypothesis. The hypothesis operationalizes and establishes the relationship of the independent and dependent variables and provides information that ultimately drives the methodologic analysis. The PICO (*patient, intervention* [or *cause*], *comparison* [if appropriate], and *outcome*) approach is reasoned, practical, and efficient (see Chapter 2).

Step 2: Accessing the Evidence

The retrieval and review of the relevant evidence is vital to ensuring the validity and success of the research. A thorough meta-analysis attempts to find published and unpublished sources of quality information. Inherent in the process of getting information into print is the risk of *publication bias* toward positive findings. It is not uncommon for studies that report nonsignificant results to remain unpublished. An important attribute of the meta-analysis is that it is inclusive of all research that meets the established criteria. Unpublished dissertations, theses, and reports may prove to be important sources of information yet difficult to track and access. Discussions with acknowledged experts in the domain can often provide a fertile and efficient source of access to these materials.

The meta-analysis lives (and dies!) by the notion of "garbage in, garbage out." It is thus incumbent that the researcher establish stringent criteria for study inclusion in the meta-analysis. A highly systematic approach to evidence retrieval and filtering (acceptance or rejection in the meta-analysis) is then performed. The established criteria (eg, RCT, sufficient power, use of valid measurement tools, appropriate use of statistics, and excellent follow-up) must be strictly adhered to and meticulously described in the final write-up. The primary risk inherent in unsystematic, narrative reviews is that there is great opportunity for bias in the retrieval, analysis, and critique of selected articles and reports. Synthesis can be substantially influenced by prior beliefs and the intent of the reviewer. When properly conducted, the meta-analysis overcomes these risks, producing an unbiased synthesis of the extant literature.

The meta-analysis is a complex undertaking, and only the general, computational themes of the meta-analysis are presented herein. As noted previously, a common metric, usually in the form of an *effect size*, is sought. A study that reported a *P* value based on a *t*-test calculation is a much different entity from a study reporting an *r* value based on a test of correlation. Instead, the researcher's task is to search for an effect size measure that provides insight into the direction and the magnitude of the intervention or interventions under study. A number of effect size measures (see Chapter 5) are available to researchers who perform a meta-analysis. A partial list of effect size measures is given in **Table 7.1**.

Table 7.1. Examples of Effect Size Measures Used in a Meta-analysis

Measure	Attributes
Cohen *d*	Difference between 2 means divided by the SD of either group; works when the variances of the 2 groups are homogeneous. In a meta-analysis, the mean differences are subtracted such that the resultant difference is positive in the direction of improvement. Measurements must be on a continuous scale. Variations exist for data using similar or different measures. Generally, effect size is as follows: *d* = 0.2, small; *d* = 0.5, medium; *d* = 0.8, large.
Correlation measures	Many types, such as phi (ϕ), *r*, point biserial, and Kendall tau (τ), depending on the nature of the variables; portray the strength of association between factors under consideration and outcome.
Number needed to treat (NNT)	Useful measure of an intervention's effectiveness. Describes the active treatment and control/comparison in achieving the desired outcome. NNT = 1 implies a favorable outcome in every patient given the treatment and no patient in the comparison group. An NNT of 50 implies that 50 patients must receive the treatment for one of them to experience the desired treatment.
Number needed to harm	Similar to NNT; used to examine adverse effect of an intervention.
Odds ratio (OR)	The probability of an event in one group compared with the probability of that event in another. If the OR = 1.0, the likelihood is the same; if the OR is > 1.0, the event is more likely in the first group. The calculation puts the odds in the experimental group in the numerator and the odds in the comparison group in the denominator.
Relative risk	The risk of an event happening in a group exposed to a treatment compared with the risk in a nonexposed group. A number > 1.0 implies greater risk.
Confidence interval (CI)	Defines a range of values likely to include a measure, generally reported as a 95% CI; implies that in 19 times of 20, the "true" value will be in the specified range of values. Many outcome measures, including those listed here, are often reported with their associated 95% CI.

Step 3: Data Synthesis and Structuring the Research Report

Once a well-executed SR is performed and the data are analyzed, the findings are synthesized and displayed. A common manner of displaying the data is to use a pictorial representation such as a forest plot and a summary effect size measure such as with an odds ratio. The forest plot displays the results of individual studies, often shown as squares, as point estimates of the mean result of each study. A horizontal line runs through each square, revealing its 95% confidence interval boundaries. The overall estimate of the treatment effect revealed by the meta-analysis and its confidence interval is found at the bottom of the plot, usually depicted as a diamond. The center of the diamond represents the pooled point estimate, and its horizontal tips or its associated line represents the confidence interval. Significance is achieved at the set level if the diamond is clear of the central line of no effect. Generally at the bottom of the forest plot is a line indicative of the odds ratio that reveals the overall magnitude of the effect (positive or negative), grounding it in clinically practical perspective (**Figure 7.2**).

The forest plot allows readers to see at a glance the information from the individual studies pooled into the meta-analysis. It provides a visual representation of the amount of variation in the results of the included studies and an estimate of the overall result based on the aggregated included studies. Forest plots are quite common in biomedical journals; their use has been greatly influenced by their widespread use in The Cochrane Collaboration (see Chapter 8).

Once the data have been analyzed, a synthesis process and the written report are begun. Consideration is given at all times to the issue of bias (see the next section), and alternative explanations or analyses are considered throughout this process. The final preparation of the report not only reiterates the original objectives of the SR but also provides a detailed description of the method that includes study inclusion criteria and justifies exclusionary criteria so that readers can more carefully assess for the influence of bias. A final, critical summary of the review process and recommendations for patient care conclude the report. **Table 7.2** is a sequential overview of the quantitative SR, or the meta-analysis.

Figure 7.2. Typical Forest Plot

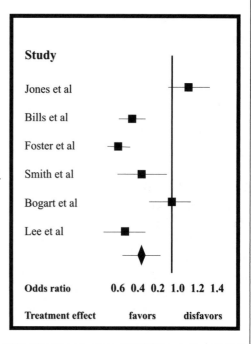

Assume a meta-analysis of the effect of a drug in preventing tachycardia. 6 studies met criteria, 4 showing effectiveness, 1 showing no effect, 1 showing a negative effect, and 1 no effect on the outcome of interest. Squares note the mean effect seen in each study, horizontal lines note the 95% CI. The vertical line is the line of no effect.

The OR is the outcome (tachycardia) in the presence of the drug; OR < 1, a favorable effect; OR = 1, no effect; OR > 1, unfavorable effect. The ♦ is the overall pooled estimate (favorable in this case) and its OR.

Abbreviations: CI, confidence interval; OR, odds ratio.

Table 7.2. Steps in the Quantitative Systematic Review Process

1. List the objectives of the planned review of the randomized control trials.
2. Carefully describe the eligibility criteria for inclusion in the systematic review.
3. Seek research that meets the stated eligibility criteria.
4. Assess each trial or published source individually for its methodologic worth.
5. Assemble the best evidence with oversight (ensuring agreement for inclusion).
6. Analyze the assembled evidence using standard statistical procedures.
7. Compare other analyses, if available.
8. Write up the critical appraisal, carefully describing the above elements, defining conclusions, and indicating potential applications to the care of patients.

A Caution: Disadvantages of the Systematic Review

Like any human enterprise, the SR is not perfect. A classic example follows. Low back pain and sciatica are common afflictions, and a great deal of research has been directed at determining the optimal treatment strategy. Two SRs published in the same year that focused on this pain complex yielded conflicting conclusions.[9] On close examination, each SR shared the same objectives and carefully included studies that met the particular inclusion criteria but differed somewhat in the judgment of quality of studies for inclusion and in the manner in which the evidence was summed up. In addition, the choice of statistic for reporting the findings resulted in one of the SRs reporting much stronger conclusions about effectiveness than the other SR. Here is a situation in which the SR itself included an element of judgment and, thus, bias.

Another classic example is found in the study of the effects of passive smoking.[10] Here it was revealed, perhaps not surprisingly, that the associated health effects described were strongly associated with the industry and funding affiliations of the researchers themselves. Researchers with tobacco industry–affiliated reviews were much more likely to report that passive smoking was not harmful.

Not everyone wholeheartedly embraces the meta-analysis. Major objections to the meta-analysis and SR can be organized into 3 general categories:

1. The potential to combine studies of great variance in overall quality
2. A possible failure on the researcher's behalf to fully consider variations in subjects, methods, interventions, or outcomes measurement
3. A nonlinear effect of the intervention—a limit (above or below) in which one factor has little or no effect on the other

Careful reading and thoughtful analysis of any published article, whether a case report, a retrospective review, an RCT, or an SR, is a responsibility each reader must assume before making direct application of findings to a patient. Evidence-based decision making does not pivot uniquely on any one published source or voice. The burden is on individual providers in the unique patient circumstance to navigate the best possible course of action.

Summary and Conclusion

The meta-analysis is supplanting the traditional narrative review as a way of describing and summarizing the evidence related to patient care intervention. The traditional narrative review is subject to many pitfalls, including bias of the authors of the selected articles and reports, the tendency for many authors to overrely on secondary (eg, textbook) sources, and bias of the authors of the narrative review. The meta-analysis represents applying the same level of systematic research rigor when reviewing the evidence as, ideally, was in place at the time that the original, cited research was performed. Combining (aggregating) and quantitatively analyzing the pooled data using a common statistical metric empowers researchers to achieve more precise estimates of the size (magnitude) of any interventional effect that might be present.

A high-quality meta-analysis provides many benefits, including the following:

- A valid and weighted course of action based on aggregated studies
- Reduced overall risk of bias
- Estimation precision and effect size of an intervention in a defined patient group
- Transparency in the overall process improving risk-benefit in a unique patient

For a rich source of high-quality meta-analyses, I recommend accessing The Cochrane Library (http://www.cochrane.org; see Chapter 8) as a starting point in search of evidence.

References

1. Dexter F, Tinker JH. Comparisons between desflurane and isoflurane or propofol on time to following commands and time to discharge: a metaanalysis. *Anesthesiology*. 1995;83(1):77-82.

2. Brimacombe J. The advantages of the LMA over the tracheal tube or facemask: a meta-analysis. *Can J Anesth*. 1995;42(11):1017-1023.

3. Boivin JF. Risk of spontaneous abortion in women occupationally exposed to anaesthetic gases: a meta-analysis. *Occup Environ Med*. 1997;54(8):541-548.

4. Dahl JB, Jeppesen IS, Jorgensen H, Wetterslev J, Møiniche S. Intraoperative and postoperative analgesic efficacy and adverse effects of intrathecal opioids in patients undergoing cesarean section with spinal anesthesia: a qualitative and quantitative systematic review. *Anesthesiology*. 1999;91(6):1919-1927.

5. Block BM, Liu SS, Rowlingson AJ, Cowan AR, Cowan JA Jr, Wu CL. Efficacy of postoperative epidural analgesia: a meta-analysis. *JAMA*. 2003;290(18):2455-2463.

6. Cheng DC, Bainbridge D, Martin JE, Novich RJ; and the Evidence-Based Perioperative Clinical Outcomes Research Group. Does off-pump coronary artery bypass reduce mortality, morbidity, and resource utilization when compared with conventional coronary artery bypass? A meta-analysis of randomized trials. *Anesthesiology*. 2005;102(1):188-203.

7. Kuratani N, Oi Y. Greater incidence of emergence agitation in children after sevoflurane anesthesia as compared with halothane: a meta-analysis of randomized controlled trials. *Anesthesiology*. 2008;109(2):225-232.

8. Biddle C. Meta-analysis of the effectiveness of nonsteroidal anti-inflammatory drugs in a standardized pain model. *AANA J*. 2002;70(2):111-114.

9. Hopayian K, Mugford M. Conflicting conclusions from two systematic reviews of epidural steroid injections for sciatica: which evidence should general practitioners heed? *Br J Gen Pract*. 1999;49(438):57-61.

10. Barnes DE, Bero LA. Why review articles on the health effects of passive smoking reach different conclusions. *JAMA*. 1998;279(19):1566-1570.

CHAPTER EIGHT

A Brief Introduction and Overview of The Cochrane Collaboration

Archie Cochrane was a remarkable man. A British physician-epidemiologist, he served during World War II, was captured, and managed, as best he could, the healthcare needs of a battalion-sized group of allied prisoners under conditions of severe deprivation and unspeakable horror. When he reentered the civilian sector, he pioneered—in the spirit of the father of epidemiology, John Lund—approaches to the provision of healthcare that were to prove prescient. In 1972, he wrote a book in which he observed, "It is surely a great criticism of our profession that we have not organized a critical summary, by specialty or subspecialty, adapted periodically, of all relevant randomized controlled trials."[1] This book received only marginal attention in its time, but we now recognize it as capturing a fundamental tenet of evidence-based practice and evidence-based decision making. For his work and influence, The Cochrane Collaboration (CC) was formed and so named in 1993.

The notion of providing the latest healthcare information of high merit to healthcare providers worldwide is what the CC is all about. The CC synthesizes and makes readily available systematic reviews of healthcare interventions and promotes research designed not only to update existing reviews but also to develop systematic reviews in areas of need. The primary output of the CC is what is known as The Cochrane Database of Systematic Reviews.

The start-up collaboration of 1993 has evolved into a resource with international input and contributions from many thousands of individuals and a host of globally diverse organizations. Teams of impartial reviewers collaborate to prepare and maintain the archived reviews and ensure that only the most valid and reliable information is provided based on a standard of rigor that has come to define the excellence of the CC. The CC makes available highly organized, systematically prepared, diverse sources of reliable and valid clinical research formation that can be brought to bear on healthcare decision making.

The Cochrane Logo/Icon

The graphic icon for the CC is shown in **Figure 8.1**. It is symbolic of an early voyage in real evidence-based practice and is deserving of explanation. Each of the horizontal lines

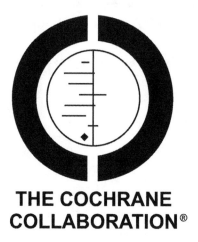

Figure 8.1. The Cochrane Collaboration Logo

THE COCHRANE
COLLABORATION®

See text for explanation.

(Reprinted with permission from The Cochrane Collaboration.)

represents the 95% confidence interval of an outcome measure resulting from a trial; the mean finding would be at each bar's midline point; the narrower the line, the tighter the confidence interval. The referenced trials are listed in chronological order from top to bottom by their date of publication (oldest at the top). The central vertical line indicates no effect, that is, if there was no effect of the intervention seen within a particular trial, its representative horizontal bar would overlap this central vertical line. Trials that demonstrated a positive or negative effect would have their representative horizontal lines placed to the left or to the right, respectively, of the center line. A diamond placed at the bottom of the diagram indicates the summary, overall effect of the representative intervention or interventions demonstrated by the included trials.

The CC icon (see Figure 8.1) depicts 7 randomized controlled trials (RCTs) that involved the administration of corticosteroids to women who were at risk of premature delivery. It had been suggested by some that administering these agents to pregnant women at risk of premature delivery might reduce the high rate of mortality and other major complications that affected the preterm infants. In 1972, the first RCT of this intervention was performed. This trial is represented by the horizontal bar at the top of the figure, here depicted as having a positive effect. A total of 7 trials (note that 7 horizontal lines depicting the trials are on the graph) were performed, and the overall effect (a positive one) is summarized by the diamond at the bottom on the graph. After this trial, many other trials revealed that the complications of immaturity (including death) could be reduced 30% to 50% with this intervention. Because the trials were small and not well communicated, this simple, highly effective intervention was not very well appreciated in the obstetric community. This was in the era before the meta-analysis was pioneered and represents a classic example of how a meta-analysis could have prevented an enormous amount of human suffering. The CC icon is known as a forest plot; the forest plot was discussed in Chapter 7 (see Figure 7.2).

Exploring and Using The Cochrane Library

The CC contains a wealth of material, including databases, journals, online books, reference works, and even podcasts. Its rich source of systematic reviews, as well as individual RCTs if a systematic review is not currently available on a topic, can be accessed by simply visiting the website. The CC houses what is essentially a virtual library and is generally referred to as The Cochrane Library. The Cochrane Library continues to evolve in part because the science of data analysis, evaluation, and retrieval is not static; rather, it too is advancing as new methods and approaches come to light. Visiting the site at http://www.cochrane.org gains you admission to amazingly diverse, logically organized RCTs and systematic reviews that can be accessed with ease and at no cost (**Figure 8.2**). Users requiring more information than the abstracts and summaries provide can access the full-text reviews by paid subscription, on a pay-per-view basis, or by departmental or institutional license.

Time Considerations and The Cochrane Library

A primary objective of the CC is getting the latest and most valid information to clinicians, recognizing that clinicians are under considerable time and production constraints in maintaining currency with respect to the latest literature. As noted, The Cochrane Library is in constant evolution, and, as of this late 2012 writing, there are well over 500,000 clinical trials in its database, a number that far exceeds MEDLINE's contingent.

Once at the Cochrane homepage, a wide variety of options are available for easy access. For example, for a scheduled case involving aortic surgery, an anesthesia provider wants an update on epidural vs parenteral opioids for pain management. Having the latest and most valid evidence empowers anesthetists to confidently discuss options with patients and fine-tune overall management plans. Figure 8.2 is the CL homepage from which you can access an enormous and diverse range of clinically relevant evidence summaries.

One component of the CC that is of particular (but not exclusive) interest to nurse anesthetists is the Cochrane Anaesthesia Review Group that became active in early 2000. Because the domain of anesthesia care draws on and interacts with so many other domains, the reviews organized under this review group include anesthesia, perioperative medicine, intensive care, resuscitation, and emergency medicine. The Cochrane Anaesthesia Review Group currently draws on tens of thousands of clinical trials (and the number is growing), with brief summary evaluations of the evidence to facilitate use by clinicians and scholars and investigators alike. Clicking on "Our reviews" in the Cochrane Anaesthesia Group page (http://carg.cochrane.org) provides an alphabetized full listing of relevant search phrases. Scrolling through the list leads to the phrase "Epidural pain relief versus systemic opioid-based pain relief for abdominal aortic surgery".

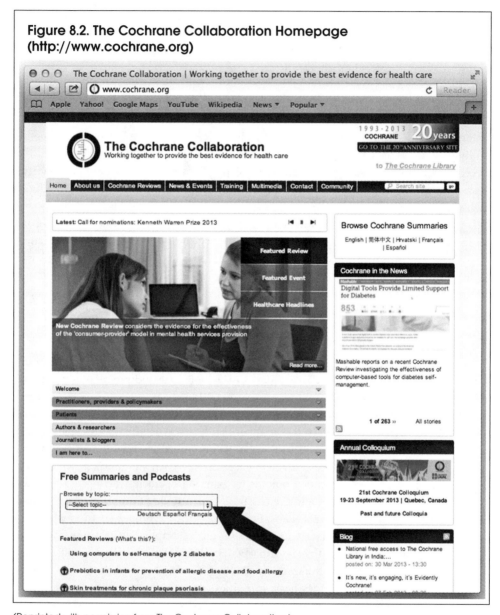

Figure 8.2. The Cochrane Collaboration Homepage (http://www.cochrane.org)

(Reprinted with permission from The Cochrane Collaboration.)

Clicking on this phrase provides a plain-language summary of the latest clinical trials related to the search phrase and an abstract that includes the following:

- Background information
- Study objectives

- Criteria for including studies in the review
- The search method
- The review method
- A description of the included studies
- The methodologic quality of the included studies
- Results
- A discussion of the findings with relevant application

Major benefits of The Cochrane Library are that it not only presents the evidence currently available on the selected topic but also describes the methodologic quality of the included trials so that users can place a value on its applicability to their current patient or patient group. Because of the logical arrangement, user-friendliness, and concise preparation that represent hallmarks of The Cochrane Library, gaining the needed information can easily be accomplished in 10 minutes or less.

Summary and Final Thoughts

It is now commonly acknowledged that the CC produces reviews that are comparable to or of better quality than reviews published in the most highly rated printed journals, and they are updated more frequently. The fundamental mission of the CC is to provide systematic reviews that are up to date and available to healthcare providers as soon as possible. The Cochrane Library is available to users worldwide and has had a key role in developing and implementing clinical practice guidelines domestically and internationally. Not only has the CC greatly improved access to clinically valuable information, but it also has been at the forefront in the research, development, and implementation of important methodologic advances. Two notable examples of this include the development of robust and sensitive search strategies for RCTs and scientific validation that conclusively revealed that failure to conceal randomization allocation was associated with bias in clinical trials.[2,3]

Having used the CC for many years, I am impressed with the improvements that I continue to encounter. In the early years, electronically accessing the reviews was not always a user-friendly experience, and even reading the reviews often proved challenging because they seemed written more for academics than for clinicians. This is no longer the case. In addition, early in its history, the CC was often remiss in not assessing the harm of certain healthcare interventions; this oversight has been corrected as well. Most recently, the CC has expanded its domain of evidentiary resources to include a wide range of important databases, including the following:

- Database of abstracts of reviews by non-Cochrane reviewers
- Central register of RCTs, allowing increased ease in finding specific trials
- Method registry of work that reports on methods used in conducting trials
- Health technology assessment database examining quality and cost-effectiveness
- Economic evaluation database to optimize research targeting cost-effectiveness

Further exploration of the CC finds tutorials; podcasts; full-text reviews; specialized domains designed and focused for clinicians, researchers, and policy makers; and even a place for patients to access information. Nurse anesthetists will find a wealth of evidence available for clinical application by visiting the CC at http://www.cochrane.org. So what are you waiting for?

References

1. Cochrane A. *Effectiveness and Efficiency: Random Reflections on Health Services.* London, England: Nuffield Provincial Hospital Trust; 1972.

2. Lefebvre C, Clarke MJ. Identifying randomized trials. In: Eggar M, Davey Smith G, Altman DG, eds. *Systematic Reviews in Health Care: Meta-analysis in Context.* London, England: BMJ Publishing; 2001:69-86.

3. Schulz KF, Chalmers I, Hayes RJ, Altman DG. Empirical evidence of bias: dimensions of methodological quality associated with estimates of treatment effects in controlled trials. *JAMA.* 1995;273(5):408-412.

CHAPTER NINE

Case Reports, Case Series, and Narrative Reviews: Cautionary Notes

Among the types of articles published in peer-reviewed journals, case reports, case series, and narrative reviews are all common and have become staples in the early educational and ongoing professional development of nurse anesthetists. The opportunity to vicariously experience the anesthetic management of a challenging patient by reading about how others dealt with the case has the potential not only to educate anesthesia providers but also to promote patient safety by avoiding pitfalls previously encountered and managed by others. Likewise, review articles serve an important purpose, providing an economical approach to managing a daunting amount of material in a concise and organized manner. In this case, someone has done all the fetching, analysis, organization, and writing, and readers are left only with the task of consuming the information.

Despite their prevalence and usefulness, there are concerns with each of these forms of informational conveyance that must be considered to maximize their value and minimize their potential drawbacks. What follows is a critique of these forms of information provision that are often used in the evidence-based decision-making process.

Case Reports and Case Series

For purposes here, these 2 forms of reports are considered together. A *case report* generally describes a procedural or pharmacologic intervention that a patient has undergone, or it may report a complication, successful outcome, or otherwise interesting or rare event. A *case series* describes a group of similar patients with one or more of the defining purposes noted for the single case report.

The use of heparin and a known complication provide the basis for an example. Heparin is commonly used in hospitalized patients. Heparin-induced thrombocytopenia with thrombosis is a known complication of heparin therapy and one that is readily diagnosed with laboratory and clinical cues. Among these are a massive decrease in the platelet count following heparin exposure, thromboembolic phenomena, resolution of the low platelet count following heparin cessation, and the detection of heparin-dependent antibodies.[1] A good deal of what we know about this complication comes from case reports and case series that describe its epidemiology, pathophysiology, and management.

Nuttal et al,[2] for instance, reported their experience with 12 patients with heparin-induced thrombocytopenia with thrombosis. Their case series described the anesthetic management of patients who underwent cardiac surgery with cardiopulmonary bypass using a standardized anesthetic protocol that included the use of hirudin as an alternative to heparin in at-risk patients. The authors meticulously detailed the case management and associated outcomes.

Do case reports and case series constitute sufficient evidence to provide the basis for future interventional choices? This question does not have a black-and-white answer. If a series is large enough (and a sample or case series size can itself be a contentious issue) and the results are "all or none"—total success or total failure—there may be justification for using the report as a reasonable form of evidence. Although it is rare to find a clinical challenge previously associated with significant adverse events or total failure that improved dramatically in a large set of patients whose management was detailed in a case series, the authors' conclusions should be viewed more positively.

The article by Nuttal et al[2] has major shortcomings. First, some patients described in the series may not have been at risk of heparin-induced thrombocytopenia with thrombosis. The diagnostic test used by the authors (enzyme-linked immunosorbent assay) has a significant rate of false-positive reporting. Comorbidities, such as renal and hepatic dysfunction, not only affect hirudin clearance but also, in general, were poorly controlled for and may make the patients in the series by Nuttal et al[2] quite different from patients who might be encountered in other situations. Intraoperative cell salvage was not used, despite a noteworthy bloody operative course, which may not reflect the type of patient care that is provided in some institutions. Issues of control, patient selection, and external validity abound.

Lack of a Control Group

Case reports and case series lack a control or comparison group, although some reports may use historical controls, a weak form of comparison due to the multitude of factors that are likely to differentiate the patients in the historical group from patients in the current group. In addition, a wide range of different management factors likely prevails. Case reports and case series are valuable for describing approaches and management decisions when the interventions are reported with exquisite care and outcomes are systematically measured. When so designed, such reports may illuminate previously darkened terrain, can generate informed clinical discussion, and can serve the extremely valuable purpose of generating focused research questions and hypotheses for subsequent study.

Potential for Bias

The risk of bias is high in case reports and case series. Because such reports lack randomization or a comparison group and because a particular outcome may or may not occur as a result of the described intervention or interventions, extreme caution is required if applying the reported interventions directly to future patients. In addition, authors of case reports and series tend to import substantial preformed opinions into their reports, and what works in their hands may not fully translate to other situations. Observer bias can be especially high because the usual absence of blinding and randomization likely helps promote outcomes that the authors embrace. Furthermore, publication bias tends to favor positive findings in general, with negative results rarely reaching a journal's final printed pages.

What Are We Left to Conclude?

Summary points about case reports and series are as follows:

- Numerous types of bias prevail.
- Results in one setting may not transfer to another.
- Because of the absence of control, the reported outcome or outcomes may not be fully related to the intervention or interventions.
- In reports of drug therapy, a placebo effect must at least be considered.
- If used, historical controls represent a poor comparison group that is prone to a host of shortcomings.
- Journal publication bias favors positive findings and outcomes.

The Narrative Review

In Chapter 7 of this book, the systematic review was described as a rich and valuable source of information for making evidence-based decisions. The narrative review is something quite different and all too often is merely a "round-up" review. Consider the image of a cowboy rounding up cattle, gathering them in—although expert in horsemanship and herding—in a somewhat arbitrary manner. Likewise, the architect of a narrative review may not report or even use a set of systematic and defined criteria to select the works cited in the review. This absence of systematically described and applied criteria for article selection provides a wealth of opportunity for bias.

Importance of Narrative Reviews

Student registered nurse anesthetists, practitioners, and academics rely heavily on the narrative review as an important source of information. Narrative reviews consolidate a large amount of information on a topic in a convenient, economical, and organized manner. Consider the review by Welliver and Cheek[3] in the *AANA Journal* on sugammadex, a novel cyclodextrin that terminates the effect of certain neuromuscular blocking drugs. The authors update readers on the pharmacology of sugammadex, include the findings of many clinical trials and dose-response studies, and offer important findings relevant to a diverse range of patients. The information provided was based on an exhaustive literature review, which would likely prove daunting for an average clinician but fulfills an essential role in defining the potential applications of a new drug and fostering its safe use.

The article by Welliver and Cheek was valuable, timely, and scholarly. The authors commendably cited each study's clinical trial phase, the number and type of subjects included in the studies, the type of anesthesia used, the dose of sugammadex used, and the observed adverse effects. However, many of the cited studies did not involve randomization, adverse events were not uniformly reported by all included studies, and methodologic issues in many studies complicate the findings. Furthermore, the concluding paragraph of the narrative review includes editorialization by selectively citing the opinions of authors whose work was cited. In addition, the primary author of the study disclosed a financial relationship with the company that produces sugammadex.[3]

The cited drawbacks are not meant to detract from the worth of the review, but they illustrate the potential for bias in what may be a roundup of cited articles that commonly constitute the narrative review. Although I would argue that the narrative review is an important mechanism to disseminate valuable and clinically relevant information, it is essential that readers critically evaluate what is presented before applying that information to the care of patients.

Risk of Bias in Narrative Reviews

Several considerations are important when judging narrative reviews. How did the author go about selecting or retrieving the included references? What about the use of primary (original studies) vs secondary (generally textbook) sources? What about the process and nature of the critique and analysis that the author performs in describing the methods and conclusions of the cited studies? What about websites (often not peer reviewed) that authors use as reference sources? Are the opinions of other authors cited in a review? Is editorializing a reason for concern?

These questions are important and often not easily answered. The authors of narrative reviews may be experts in their own right and draw on work that supports their own views. Likewise, students or nonexperts who are developing narrative reviews to enlighten or extend appreciation for a particular topic or domain of interest may, because of their own inexperience or bias, draw on sources of information that may not represent a sufficiently balanced view.

What Are We Left to Conclude?

Below are summary points about narrative reviews:

- Review articles usually lack explicit criteria for the work that is cited.
- They are subject to low methodologic quality.
- Authors may have a view they want to promote.
- The risk of readers drawing incomplete or inaccurate conclusions may be high.
- If there is insufficient evidence that included articles did not meet reasonable inclusion criteria, the report should be considered low in quality of evidence.

What Are the Alternatives?

What has been argued throughout this book is that it is important to favor randomized controlled trials and systematic reviews (including meta-analyses) in marshaling evidence important to patient care-related decision making. A checklist that can be used to determine the worth of a narrative review appears in **Table 9.1**.

Table 9.1. Quick Appraisal Tool to Judge a Review Article

Did the author seem to obtain *all* relevant studies that deal with the topic at hand?

Did the author establish and report criteria (inclusion and exclusion) for the cited studies?

Do those criteria include population attributes and size; study method, including blinding and randomization; and appropriate outcome measures?

Was there an overall rating (evaluation) of the quality of cited articles?

Was there a final—and balanced—summary of the evidence?

Was there any evidence of editorialization or conflict of interest on behalf of the authors of the narrative review?

Closing Remarks

Case reports, case series, and narrative reviews are common publication entities that are found in even the best journals. Despite their widespread use, they often have substantial limitations, especially bias, that markedly limit their value in the direct application of their findings or recommendations to an evidence-based decision-making process. It is important to appreciate that only the most stringently applied methods and findings can safely and effectively move anesthesia care toward desired perianesthetic outcomes.

References

1. Ballard JO. Anticoagulant-induced thrombosis. *JAMA.* 1999;282(4):310-312.

2. Nuttall GA, Oliver WC, Santrach PJ, et al. Patients with a history of type II heparin-induced thrombocytopenia with thrombosis requiring cardiac surgery with cardiopulmonary bypass: a prospective observational case series. *Anesth Analg.* 2003;96(2):344-350.

3. Welliver M, Cheek D. An update on sugammadex sodium. *AANA J.* 2009;77(3):219-228.

CHAPTER TEN

Will Following the Tenets of Evidence-Based Practice Improve Patient Safety? What's the Evidence?

Throughout this book, a case has been made for using evidence-based decision making (EBDM) in everyday clinical practice. Is there evidence that evidence-based practice improves care? Certainly, healthcare workers have long appreciated that the provision of services is a challenging and risky enterprise. The rather dramatic public awakening to this state of affairs came with the publication of the Institute of Medicine report, *To Err is Human,* revealing an annual rate of medical- and nursing-related patient injury exceeding 1 million per year and perhaps 100,000 deaths per year.[1] Addressing this sobering revelation has become a national priority.

Poor outcomes at the hands of healthcare workers are not always a result of human error. Although it seems obvious that healthcare interventions be based on the latest, high-grade scientific research, it is clear that too often many of the interventions that patients receive are solely experience-driven or opinion-based. If the latest and best evidence is "married" to motivated and highly qualified healthcare workers, does it not logically follow that patient safety will improve? Consider the enormous complexity of the landscape for the provision of healthcare (**Figure 10.1**). Marshaling evidence to our decision-making process will help us choose the right course.

It is well recognized that the provision of anesthesia services nationwide is iconic in the realm of patient safety. There are many reasons for this, including aggressive campaigns by the American Association of Nurse Anesthetists and the American Society of Anesthesiologists that have prioritized patient safety, the development of monitors that target specific safety issues, advances in pharmacology, greater oversight by accrediting bodies, and widespread improvements in the education and training of providers.

Has evidence-based practice increasingly found a foothold in anesthetic practice? One study revealed that most anesthetic interventions were evidence-based, although this study focused on a unique practice situation and its generalizability is thus limited.[2] My own reading of the literature, observation of practice patterns nationwide, listening to countless lectures at a wide range of conferences, and discussions with clinicians across the country suggest that practice patterns, interventional approaches, and local standards of care vary considerably. These findings lead me to believe that evidence-based practice is inconsistently embraced.

96 **CHAPTER TEN**

Will Following the Tenets of Evidence-Based Practice Improve Patient Safety? What's the Evidence?

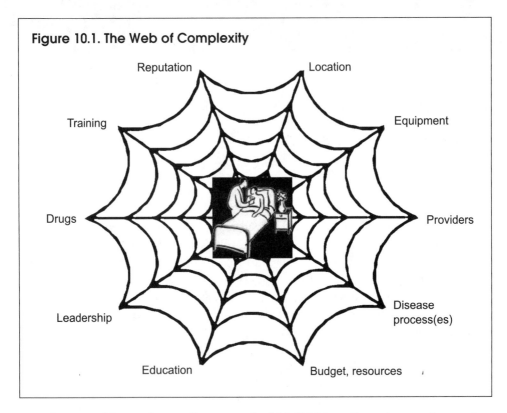

Figure 10.1. The Web of Complexity

In the general hospital care of patients, the 100,000 Lives Campaign stands as a dramatic testimonial to the tangible rewards associated with adherence to evidence-based care supplanting individual provider-variant care.[3] This program was a tangible response to the Institute of Medicine's report just mentioned[1] (**Figure 10.2**). Approximately 2,300 hospitals across the United States implemented 6 evidence-based, lifesaving interventions, resulting in the saving of 122,300 lives during the study period.[4] This landmark study used valid and reliable measures to track the successes and failures associated with each of the 6 interventions. The selected interventions were based on strong, multidimensional evidence and were judged feasible and practical to implement. The interventions applied were the following:

- Prevention of central venous line infection
- Prevention of surgical site infection
- Prevention of ventilator-associated pneumonia
- Use of rapid response teams
- Standardized care for myocardial infarction
- Prevention of adverse drug events during transfer of care

CHAPTER TEN   97

Will Following the Tenets of Evidence-Based Practice Improve Patient Safety? What's the Evidence?

Figure 10.2. The 100,000 Lives Campaign in the Wake of the Institute of Medicine's Report, *To Err is Human*

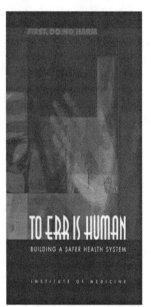

The 100,000 Lives Campaign was a nationwide initiative launched by the Institute for Healthcare Improvement (IHI) in an effort to significantly reduce morbidity and mortality in the American healthcare system. Building on the successful work of healthcare providers all over the world, a select group of best practices were embraced to help participating hospitals extend or save as many as 100,000 lives.

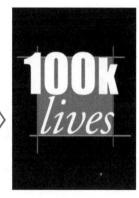

The 100K Lives Campaign was inspired by the challenges posed in the Institute of Medicine's report.

In the wake of this milestone effort, entirely grounded in the principles of evidence-based practice and EBDM, hospitals nationwide have come to recognize that the guidelines established in this effort have led to consequential differences in the efficacy and safety of care provided to hospitalized patients. Based on this early success, the Institute for Healthcare Improvement initiated the Five Million Lives Campaign, whose goal is to enroll 4,000 hospitals nationwide with the goal of preventing 5 million incidents of medically related harm to patients, using 12 evidence-based interventions.

A milestone article published in 1991 revealed that about 4% of all hospitalized patients experienced an iatrogenic injury, including death.[5] On closer examination of the adverse events, two-thirds were viewed as preventable (errors in treatment provided)

98   CHAPTER TEN

Will Following the Tenets of Evidence-Based Practice Improve Patient Safety? What's the Evidence?

and, thus, potentially manageable by error-reduction strategies. There is even more recent evidence that nosocomial infections (ie, hospital-acquired) are occurring at a rate not previously seen and may affect upward of 10% of all hospitalized patients, with a significant associated mortality.[6,7] This rate increase may largely be the result of inconsistent asepsis, especially the simple failure of healthcare providers to wash their hands between patient interventions. Here is another sobering reality: medication errors are responsible for more deaths in the United States than AIDS, breast cancer, and motor vehicle accidents.[8] I believe that many adverse (including lethal) events currently considered impossible to manage or unpreventable given our current level of scientific knowledge will be potentially manageable by future advances in our cognitive base via research.

Recent examples of evidence-based "success stories" abound. A partial list follows:

- Protocols to reduce ventilator-associated pneumonia
- Maximal sterile barrier use during insertion of central venous lines
- Focused nutritional intervention in postsurgical and critically ill patients
- Antibiotic prophylaxis to reduce surgical site infection
- Ultrasound guidance during placement of central lines
- Full-time intensivists in intensive care units
- Computerization and clinical decision support to reduce medication errors
- Pressure-relieving bedding materials to reduce pressure ulcers
- Greater use of regional over general anesthesia in obstetric delivery
- Nonpharmacologic approaches to the treatment of postoperative nausea and vomiting
- Intrathecal opiates in perioperative pain management
- Technological advances, such as cerebral oxygen monitors, noninvasive cardiac output monitors, and positron emission tomography scans
- Venous thromboembolism prophylaxis
- Antibiotic-impregnated central venous catheters and insertion-site dressings (eg, BioPatch, Ethicon Inc)
- Lung-protective mechanical ventilation strategies

Seduction by Authority and the Power of Big Business

Humans are not only prone to error but also may fall victim to a kind of seduction that I refer to as "collective worship at the altar of the new and improved." Drug and technology companies are in the business of making money, and their primary approach to achieving this end is to bring new products to the marketplace. So-called blockbuster drugs are good examples. "Blockbusters" are defined in the industry as drugs that generate in excess of $1 billion annually. Examples of these include certain antipsychotics, sleep aids, and type 2 cyclooxygenase inhibitors. There is substantial and ongoing controversy associated with each of these example blockbusters regarding their effectiveness in the general population and their overall safety. The manner in which drugs are aggressively marketed (directly to the public via a blitzkrieg of radio, television, and lay magazine ads urging "Ask your

CHAPTER TEN 99

Will Following the Tenets of Evidence-Based Practice Improve Patient Safety? What's the Evidence?

doctor if this is right for you") and the curious human perception that "things that cost more and are newer must somehow be better" create an environment that may result in uncritical acceptance of products without sufficient evidence to do so.

The following is a list of interventions that were once in widespread use but have been discounted as worthless or dangerous, begging the question, How could this have happened?

- Bloodletting
- Diethylstilbestrol to improve pregnancy outcome
- Thalidomide for pregnancy-related nausea
- "Twilight sleep" for labor and delivery
- Routine performance of episiotomy
- Innovar (a fixed injectable drug combination of fentanyl and droperidol)
- Enteryx device (from Boston Scientific Corp, foam injected at the gastroesophageal junction to prevent reflux)
- Chymopapain injection for herniated vertebral disk disease
- Raplon (rapacuronium bromide from Organon Inc)
- Vioxx (rofecoxib from Merck Inc)
- Atypical antipsychotic drugs for treatment of dementia
- Chiropractic manipulation for cancer, heart disease, and other major ailments
- Gastric freezing and vagotomy for treatment of peptic ulcer
- Many devices with deadly side effects removed from use by the US Food and Drug Administration in the last 5 years

The story of the "coxibs" (selective cyclooxygenase type 2 inhibitors) deserves a special notation as an example of the healthcare system gone woefully wrong. The coxibs were originally developed and approved for the treatment of patients with rheumatoid arthritis and osteoarthritis, only later becoming commonplace in the treatment of acute pain. There proved to be considerable overlap with the indications of nonselective, nonsteroidal anti-inflammatory drugs, and an unexpected bonanza marketplace suddenly appeared. The drugs were widely prescribed, seemingly creating a population of patient consumers exceeding that of regular nonsteroidal anti-inflammatory drug users.[9] Aggressive marketing, incomplete research disclosure, uncritical acceptance by healthcare providers, endorsement by third-party payers, and unreasonable public (patient) expectations combined to produce an illogical state of use that led to many unintended catastrophic and near-catastrophic outcomes.

ALLHAT: Big Study, Important Outcomes, Little Impact

The Antihypertensive and Lipid-Lowering Treatment to Prevent Heart Attack Trial (ALLHAT) was a randomized, double-blind, multicenter, clinical trial performed from February 1994 through March 2002. Given the importance of antihypertensive therapy in reducing cardiovascular-related morbidity and mortality and the uncertainty about the optimal first step in treatment, the investigators conducted a trial of 33,357 participants

100 **CHAPTER TEN**

Will Following the Tenets of Evidence-Based Practice Improve Patient Safety? What's the Evidence?

older than 54 years with hypertension and at least 1 other major risk factor. The findings were published in *JAMA*.[10]

This study was one of the largest (> 33,000 subjects) and most expensive (approximately $130 million) clinical trials ever organized by the federal government and was intended to systematically evaluate expensive vs less expensive interventions. The conclusions of this highly powered, methodically superb study were clear. Thiazide-type diuretics are superior in preventing 1 or more major forms of cardiovascular disease events, have few side effects, and are far less expensive; diuretics should be preferred for first-step antihypertensive therapy. Other findings emerged with immediate clinical practice implications, including the early finding that Cardura (doxazosin, a new α-blocker made by Pfizer) was associated with a doubling in the rate of heart failure; its use in the trial was suspended. Widespread application of the findings of this study would save the nation billions of dollars in treating tens of millions of US citizens with hypertension. The downside? The conclusions posed a major threat to companies (eg, Pfizer) that produced blockbuster antihypertensive agents. Despite initially using industry-crafted responses urging the continued use of Cardura, Pfizer stopped promoting the drug in 2000.

Initially, the overall percentage of hypertensive patients receiving diuretics increased to about 40% in the year after ALLHAT, up from 30% to 35% in the year before ALLHAT (personal communication, Dr R. Clark, VCU Medical Center, September 2012). Since then, the use of diuretics has fallen back, and overall the use of newer antihypertensive agents has grown much faster than what was initially seen with the use of diuretics.

How could such solid evidence favoring the safety and efficacy of an older, cheaper intervention over newer, more expensive interventions be ignored? In a compelling 2004 article in *JAMA*, Naylor,[11] with the benefit of systematic hindsight analysis, wrote:

> The ALLHAT investigators are trying to facilitate the translation of their findings into practice, but no team of academic clinicians can hope to match the marketing know-how and deep pockets of the pharmaceutical industry. What is needed are stronger mechanisms to avoid premature retirement of aging orphan drugs that are still useful or may have new indications.

Because of the importance of the findings and the perception that the study was not translating well to practice, the National Heart, Lung, and Blood Institute formulated a committee of the 147 ALLHAT investigators to give formal presentations nationwide to better disseminate the findings. As reported in *The New York Times,* one of the committee members, Richard Grimm Jr, MD, received approximately $200,000 from Pfizer in 2003, the year after ALLHAT's publication.[12] This obvious conflict of interest, as well as other political and scientific disagreements, ultimately led to the ALLHAT lead investigator and committee chairman, Curt Furberg, MD, resigning in frustration.

Biologicals: An Emerging Class of Drugs With Attendant Emerging Concerns

In 1982, the first of a new class of drugs, known as "biologicals," was approved for human use. This drug, recombinant insulin, has since been followed by more than 250 biological

CHAPTER TEN   101

Will Following the Tenets of Evidence-Based Practice Improve Patient Safety? What's the Evidence?

drugs. *Biologicals* are defined as drugs whose active ingredients are produced or extracted from a natural biological source. Among such agents are monoclonal antibody–based agents, a large number of vaccines, recombinant blood products, and a host of other pharmaceuticals. The market has grown enormously, demonstrated by the observation that between the years 2003 and 2006, approximately 24% of all new chemical agents approved by American regulatory authorities were biologicals.[13]

In a benchmark study, the first of its kind, investigators sought to determine the frequency and nature of safety-related regulatory interventions in approved biologicals; the findings were genuinely disturbing.[14] Approximately 25% of the widely used, new biologicals for common disorders were found to result in serious adverse effects that resulted in regulatory actions. These actions included black box warnings, direct mailings to providers warning them of risks, and mandated market withdrawals, all for patient safety reasons. Many of the adverse drug reactions were related to biologicals hindering or modulating the immune system such that infections (bacterial, viral, and fungal), blood and lymphatic system disorders, immune system disorders, and benign and malignant tumors resulted.

The issue that surrounds biologicals is the same as for other classes of drugs; the healthcare provider's comprehensive knowledge of a recently approved drug, especially regarding its safety, is simply not known. Although this may seem like a harsh and over-generalized indictment, the evidence to support it is compelling. There are many factors, discussed throughout this book, that account for this, including constraints associated with drug research. Among these constraints are sample size, sample diversity (representativeness), the nature of controlled trials, industry (and possibly investigator) bias, and aggressiveness in marketing a new product.

Communication

Communication issues between and among patients and their healthcare providers remain a common theme in the generation of safety concerns, including medical and nursing error. Communication is an enormously complex phenomenon, and many variables serve to influence it, several of which are illustrated in **Figure 10.3**.

Amid the challenges of providing healthcare, coupled with the inherent limitations of human performance, it is vital that clinicians have standardized communication tools, that they foster an environment in which individuals are empowered to speak up and express concerns, and that they share simple and well-recognized critical language elements that reliably alert team members to unsafe situations. Communication is far too often entirely situation- or personality-dependent. The evidence reveals that highly dependable, safety-conscious organizations, such as nuclear power entities, commercial aviation, and the military, that use standardized processes, tools, and behaviors have manifestly reduced risk and improved the opportunities for successfully achieving desired outcomes.[15,16] Evidence-based decision making prevails in the communication arena!

102 **CHAPTER TEN**

Will Following the Tenets of Evidence-Based Practice Improve Patient Safety? What's the Evidence?

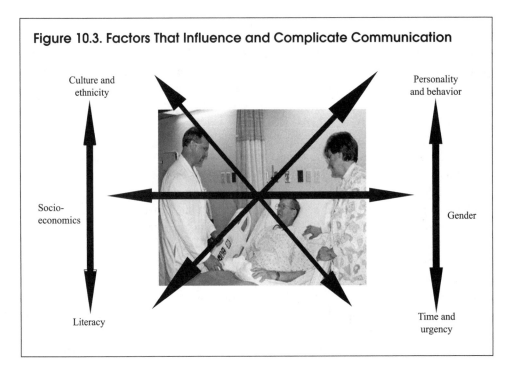

Figure 10.3. Factors That Influence and Complicate Communication

Culture and ethnicity

Personality and behavior

Socio-economics

Gender

Literacy

Time and urgency

Conclusions

A report published by the Institute for Safe Medication Practices noted that the number of serious problems, including death, linked to medications is at an all-time high.[17] Heparin and varenicline (Chantix), a drug used in helping smokers stop using tobacco by easing withdrawal symptoms, are good examples of drugs with an extremely high rate of adverse reactions. Adverse reactions that were not reported in the preliminary trials were present in the case of varenicline, with more than 1,000 reports of serious injury linked to this drug. This serves as a powerful reminder that intense "pharmacovigilance" is essential in any drug-administration procedure, no matter what the drug, because each patient is unique.

The responsibility for drug, procedural, and technological folly (leading to uncritical application to patients) is shared by many, including the manufacturer, health-related oversight organizations such as the Food and Drug Administration, journal editors, and reviewers who permit flawed or biased research to become mainstream, physicians and nurses who apply the product to patients, and patients themselves (in some cases). Clearly, better education ("academic detailing") of healthcare providers, more stringent regulation by oversight organizations, encouragement of patients to ask more questions, and the routine use of the principles of evidence-based practice and EBDM will go a long way in insulating patients from faulty, ineffective, or dangerous interventions. Just because something is new does not guarantee that it is better.

CHAPTER TEN 103

Will Following the Tenets of Evidence-Based Practice Improve Patient Safety? What's the Evidence?

Nota Bene: A Historical Milestone in Evidence-Based Anesthesia Care

Before closing this chapter, I would like to cite what appears to be the first example of evidence-based practice in the domain of anesthesiology, one that led to a major advancement in patient safety. In 1955, the venerable anesthesiologist B. R. Fink reported the findings of a study whose goal was to understand why patients often became cyanotic during recovery from general anesthesia, despite good ventilation.[18]

Fink established the purpose of the research with a brief set of clinical observations and established a framework with citations from the literature. A series of in vitro experiments followed by in vivo research led to the following evidence-based conclusion: "It is concluded that anoxia arises because the outward diffusion of nitrous oxide lowers the alveolar partial pressure of oxygen. It is suggested that this phenomenon can become a causative factor of cardiac arrest...."[16(p519)] Fink's systematic use of evidentiary principles was prescient. To this day those early recommendations rising from his work are applied daily in clinical practice.

References

1. Kohn LT, Corrigan JM, Donaldson MS, eds. *To Err is Human: Building a Safer Health System.* Washington, DC: National Academies Press; 2000.

2. Myles PS, Bain DL, Johnson F, McMahon R. Is anaesthetic practice evidence-based? *Br J Anaesth.* 1999;82(4):591-595.

3. Gosfield A, Reinertsen J. The 100,000 Lives Campaign: crystallizing standards of care for hospitals. *Health Aff.* 2005;24(6):1560-1570.

4. Thomas K, VanOyen-Force M, Rasmussen D, Dodd D, Whildin S. Rapid response team. *Crit Care Nurse.* 2007;27(1):20-27.

5. Leape LL, Brennan TA, Laird NM, et al. The nature of adverse events in hospitalized patients: results from the Harvard Medical Practice Study II. *N Engl J Med.* 1991;324(6):377-384.

6. National Nosocomial Infections Surveillance System Report: data summary from January 1992 through June 2004, issued October 2004. *Am J Infect Control.* 2004;32(8):470-485.

7. Loftus RW, Koff MD, Burchman CC, et al. Transmission of pathogenic bacterial organisms in the anesthesia work area. *Anesthesiology.* 2008;109(3):399-407.

8. Ortiz E, Meyer G, Burstin H. Clinical informatics and patient safety at the Agency for Healthcare Research and Quality. *J Am Med Inform Assoc.* 2002;9(6 suppl 1):S2-S7. doi: 10.1197/jamia.M1216.

9. Anderson GM, Juurlink D, Detsky AS. Newly approved does not always mean new and improved. *JAMA.* 2008;299(13):1598-1600.

104   CHAPTER TEN

Will Following the Tenets of Evidence-Based Practice Improve Patient Safety? What's the Evidence?

10. Furberg CD, Wright JJ, Davis BR, et al. Major outcomes in high-risk hypertensive patients randomized to angiotensin-converting enzyme inhibitor or calcium channel blocker vs diuretic: the ALLHAT. *JAMA*. 2002;288(23):2981-2997.

11. Naylor CD. The complex world of prescribing behavior. *JAMA*. 2004;291(1):104-106.

12. Pollack A. Minimal impact of a big hypertension study. *New York Times*. November 27, 2008. http://www.nytimes.com/2008/11/28/business/28govtest. html?emc=eta1. Accessed September 18, 2012.

13. Walsh G. Biopharmaceutical benchmarks 2006. *Nat Biotechnol*. 2006;24(7):769-776.

14. Giezen TJ, Mantel-Teeuwisse AK, Straus SK, Schellekens H, Leufkens HG, Egberts AC. Safety-related regulatory actions for biologicals approved in the United States and the European Union. *JAMA*. 2008;300(6):1887-1896.

15. Pronovost P, Weast B, Rosenstein B, et al. Implementing and validating a comprehensive unit-based safety program. *J Patient Safety*. 2005;1(1):33-40.

16. Leonard M, Graham S, Bonacum D. The human factor: the critical importance of effective teamwork and communication in providing safe care. *Qual Safety Health Care*. 2004;13(suppl 1):i85-i90.

17. Institute for Safe Medication Practices. Strong safety signal seen for new varenicline risks. http://www.ismp.org/docs/vareniclinestudy.asp. Accessed September 18, 2012.

18. Fink BR. Diffusion anoxia. *Anesthesiology*. 1955;16(4):511-519.

CHAPTER ELEVEN

Teaching Evidence-Based Practice and Evidence-Based Decision Making

There are many approaches to teaching, and virtually all successful educators use strategies that are hybrids of approaches they encountered in their own scholastic and professional preparation. It is not the intent of this chapter to review the many teaching and learning theories and principles relevant to classroom and clinical teaching. However, 2 works, a classic by Combs[1] and another by Marzano,[2] have proved invaluable to me during my academic career, and I briefly summarize what I believe are a few of the essential points from each of these works.

Combs[1] observed that to create an effective learning milieu, 3 characteristics are needed. These characteristics have consistently proved well suited to the domain in which we work and have great relevance to teaching evidence-based practice:

1. The atmosphere should facilitate the exploration of meaning; the learner needs to understand the risks and rewards of seeking new knowledge and understanding.
2. Frequent opportunities to confront new information and experiences must be provided in the search for meaning. Such opportunities must be provided in ways that allow students to do more than simply receive information.
3. New meaning should be acquired through a process of personal discovery. The methods used to encourage such personal discovery must be highly individualized and adapted to the learner's own style and pace for learning.

Marzano[2] makes certain assumptions about creating an effective and dynamic learning-centered environment:

1. Instruction must reflect the best of what we know about how learning occurs.
2. Learning involves a complex system of interactive processes that include the multiple dimensions of the way people learn.
3. The bulk of research demonstrates that instruction focusing on large, inter-disciplinary themes is the most effective way to promote learning.
4. Instruction should include explicit teaching of higher-level perceptions and mental habits that facilitate learning.

5. A comprehensive approach to teaching includes instruction that is teacher-directed but provides opportunities for student-directed activity.
6. Assessment should focus on the learners' use of knowledge and complex reasoning rather than their recall of low-level information.

"Doing as I Do, Rather Than Doing as I Say"

In the classroom and clinical settings, evidence-based practice has become an essential component of the professional practice of nurse anesthesia educators. One important approach to teaching the principles of evidence-based practice is for the teacher to actively engage in the process of evidence-based practice. The value inculcation that occurs in a learner who observes the teacher engaging in evidence-based decision making (EBDM) can be powerful. Seeing a teacher or mentor engage in evidence-based practice reveals humility (acknowledging that the mentor's knowledge has limits) and demonstrates a buy-in to the notion of being a lifelong learner. It also promotes the highly desirable quality of willingness to ask for assistance.

First and foremost, a faculty member who wants to teach evidence-based practice should embrace and actively use evidence-based practice in professional life. "Do as I do," is a more powerful form of value inculcation for students than "do as I say," which may occur in the absence of the actual behavior. Role modeling thus becomes an effective, practical illustration of the techniques and application of evidence-based practice. For example, a student observes her faculty mentor thoroughly explain the anesthetic options to a patient following a thorough preanesthetic assessment, obtain well-informed consent from the patient, complete a thorough preuse check of the anesthesia machine, skillfully prepare for and administer a subarachnoid block for a patient undergoing a total knee arthroplasty, and vigilantly monitor the patient throughout the case. The professional role modeling that occurs in the doing is likely associated with more long-term imprinting than if the behaviors are spelled out in the classroom but not actively used in the clinical setting.

Similarly, when the principles of evidence-based practice are embraced and used by faculty members, students see the usefulness of those principles at the point of care, where resources, technology, and knowledge are ultimately brought to bear on the care of individual patients. There is simply no substitute for "practice as I do" rather than "practice as I preach."

Practical Pointers for Teaching Evidence-Based Practice to a Student or Colleague

The following are some suggestions for what I believe to be practical ideas and approaches for teaching and instilling the worth of evidence-based practice to student registered nurse anesthetists or interested colleagues or to simply consider in your own practice.

Facilitate Asking the Right Question

Students encounter conundrums, areas of uncertainty, and fundamental clinical questions every day. When working with learners, faculty members have an opportunity to help them frame questions amenable to evidence-based inquiry and assist them in developing strategies that are responsive to these questions. By doing, so, faculty members also help themselves to implement evidence-based practice.

For example, for a patient having a total knee arthroplasty, a student's question centers on postoperative pain management. Narrowing the focus of the question makes it not only more clinically relevant but also more amenable to evidence-based inquiry. For example, the question, "What are the advantages and disadvantages of postoperative regional analgesia compared with parenteral opioids?" is a start that helps simplify the task ahead. Refinement of the question to include specific information related to the case at hand provides further, practical focus. These refinements might include consideration of specific drugs (eg, fentanyl, morphine, lidocaine, and ropivacaine), specific techniques (eg, intravenous, intramuscular, intrathecal, extradural, and interscalene techniques and patient-controlled analgesia), and specific patient information (eg, age, body habitus, and comorbidities).

The ability to ask a good question that is amenable to evidence-based inquiry is a skill that develops over time and, once achieved, should be shared with others. Use of the PICO (patient, intervention, comparison, outcome) mnemonic to develop a researchable clinical question is an excellent approach; for an in-depth discussion of the PICO approach, see Chapter 2.

Use Evidence-Based Practice for Real-World, Clinically Relevant Questions

In patient care, evidence-based practice is a process that is designed to bring the most valid and clinically applicable information to the decision-making process. By definition, it deals with real-world, practical problems faced in the anesthetic care of patients. Each day, a nurse anesthetist encounters patients with common and uncommon issues. In an average week, a nurse anesthetist is likely to encounter some or all of the following questions:

- Is a 12-lead electrocardiogram needed for a 55-year-old healthy man having a herniorrhaphy under spinal anesthesia?
- For a patient with a latex allergy, what is the optimal perioperative management?
- What is the best approach to prevent postoperative nausea and vomiting in a 35-year-old woman undergoing laparoscopic gastric banding?
- Does epidural analgesia during labor affect the obstetric outcome?
- What is the current recommendation regarding how "tightly" a diabetic patient's blood glucose level should be controlled?
- What discharge criteria are best for a patient undergoing spinal anesthesia in an ambulatory setting?
- For carotid endarterectomy, is regional anesthesia preferable to general anesthesia?
- Is regional anesthesia safe for patients taking antiplatelet medication?
- Is positive end-expiratory pressure needed for this patient?

- What are the latest recommendations regarding perioperative β-blocker use?
- Does the choice of intraoperative fluid influence postoperative outcome?
- Is it safe to proceed with a hernia repair in an afebrile, 28-month-old child with a runny nose?
- Is it safe for a patient to breastfeed after general anesthesia?
- How soon can an ambulatory surgical patient drive a car after general anesthesia with propofol, sevoflurane, and sufentanil?

Consider the following scenario that any nurse anesthetist might encounter in an average day in practice:

Assume you have a patient scheduled for a bilateral inguinal herniorrhaphy who has a history of asthma and daily use of a β-agonist inhaler, a 1 pack-per-day use of cigarettes, and combined protein C and antithrombin III deficiencies (both leading to a hypercoagulable state). The patient is afraid of needles and voices great fear of the operating room because of events he has seen on TV. Although you recognize the associated risk of thromboembolic complications in the patient and talk with the student assigned to you about the relevant concerns, you engage in a process of evidence seeking so that an optimum anesthetic plan can be pursued.

If it is the day before surgery and you have the luxury of time with the student, an extensive search of the literature using established electronic databases can be performed. In addition, you draw on your own experience and knowledge of the pathophysiology and discuss management options with colleagues to learn of their experience with and knowledge of the relevant patient issues. As the risks and benefits of various approaches are thoughtfully considered (eg, a regional vs general technique and preanesthetic administration of agents that modify the clotting cascade), the patient's perspective is brought into the discussion to actively engage him in the planning process as the options and the associated risks and benefits are described to him.

If the patient is not available the day before surgery, a plan is developed to involve the patient upon arrival on the day of surgery. Although teaching the content to the student is important, what is of equivalent importance is revealing to the student the manner in which the relevant information is obtained and how it is evaluated in the context of this particular patient in a time-efficient manner.

Throughout this process, the student is encouraged to be an active participant in gathering information or, if too "junior," is invited into the process as an active observer. When appropriate, you ask the student to respond to your questions, not to test his or her grasp of minutiae, but to help assess the student's level of understanding of the major anesthetic considerations. As the evidence is gathered and the EBDM process unfolds, the value inculcation that accompanies this process represents an educational opportunity and an essential professional responsibility of the faculty member.

If it is the day of surgery, time constraints are likely to limit the depth and extent of evidence-based research. But even in this setting, the manner in which information is obtained, such as discussion with colleagues, use of electronic tools such as PubMed clinical queries (see Chapter 2), textbook or journal use, drawing on one's own experience and knowledge, and interaction with the patient, are attended by major potential for value inculcation.

Keep the Process Practical

The use of EBDM does not require one to be a researcher or statistician. Understanding what different research methods can (and cannot) do is invaluable to the evidence-based practice process, as is the ability to interpret statistical procedures, but this does not imply that one needs to perform research or statistical analysis. Graduate programs at the master and clinical doctorate levels have requisite core courses that assist students to achieve a foundation of research comprehension. Although a research doctorate (Doctor of Philosophy) requires the performance of a substantive piece of novel research, other graduate degrees, including the master's and clinical doctorate, generally emphasize the ability to interpret and appropriately apply research findings. This latter set of skills is necessary to be a successful consumer of evidence-based practice.

Being an evidence-based nurse anesthetist does not require enormous amounts of time. For healthcare providers, evidence-based practice is designed to make the care provided safer and more effective. Evidence-based practice is not about reviewing every article, teasing out minutiae, and searching for subtle flaws in design, method, or interpretation. In teaching the underlying principles and procedures of evidence-based practice, it is essential for teachers to keep the process *connected to the patient under consideration*. Sometimes in their eagerness to teach evidence-based practice, instructors put too much onto students and, in that process, discourage future use of evidence-based practice. The principles and processes of evidence-based practice require time to think and time to absorb. Don't rush, pressure, or overwhelm those new to the domain.

Consider What Evidence-Based Practice Is and What It Is Not

Many people take issue with evidence-based practice and criticize its philosophical tenets on multiple levels. First, some criticize evidence-based practice and EBDM as a misguided attempt to substitute new research findings for tried-and-true methods. Because there is often a deficit in coherent scientific evidence, these opponents believe the process falters because of a lack of foundation. Second, others argue that it is very difficult to apply evidence to the care of individual patients. Third, still others lament the need to develop new skills. Fourth, there also, of course, is the issue of limited time and resources. Although it is important to acknowledge these concerns, my view is that they are largely misguided and largely unfounded.

Evidence-based practice is designed to complement a provider's clinical expertise and provide new and useful information that may be integrated with what the provider already knows and considers in the context of the patient's unique circumstances. I would like to briefly deal with each of the 4 aforementioned criticisms.

First, healthcare knowledge is expanding exponentially, and the gaps and knowledge deficits that exist are rapidly filling. New knowledge and practice are not intended to erase existing knowledge and practice but to complement and refine them. Second, the foundation of evidence-based practice is to take the very best information and apply it to a unique patient in the context of that patient's circumstances. Individual patient values are actively sought and incorporated into the plan of care as the patient is actively invited to participate in the decision-making process. Third, I acknowledge that it is incumbent on individual practitioners to develop new skills, especially the skills related to searching the literature electronically and becoming a more critical appraiser of what is found. As adult learners, nurse anesthetists are more than capable of acquiring the skill set necessary to be a competent evidence-based practice care provider.

Regarding the fourth issue of limited time and resources, I have indicated elsewhere in this text that I believe this is the major obstacle to actively and routinely using evidence-based practice in day-to-day clinical activities. I am optimistic, however, that this obstacle is hardly insurmountable given the wide range of readily available evidence-based resources, especially those that can be accessed electronically. Because of the nature of these resources and search tools, many of which are noted in Appendix 2.1, busy clinicians can rest assured that what they will encounter is highly relevant and valid information produced with clinicians' time constraints in mind. Of course, the responsibility lies with clinicians to ask a focused question that will lend itself to the most important issues being adequately addressed in a time-conscious manner.

Consider Making a Critically Appraised Topic Summary

Sauve et al[3] developed a tool that represents a structured summary of the evidence addressing a clinical question to facilitate learning the use of evidence-based practice; it is called a critically appraised topic summary (CATS). This type of approach to learning how to engage in an evidence-based inquiry is one that is somewhat akin to the clinical care plan, a ubiquitous part of the early training and education of nurse anesthetists.

The key components of CATS emphasize its "summary" rather than "comprehensive" nature, as follows:

- Statement of the purpose
- Name of the reviewer
- Date of completion of the CATS
- A well-constructed question (ideally just 1, but possibly 2)
- Indication of the search strategies used
- Brief description of the evidence retrieved
- Critical, balanced appraisal
- Important conclusions directed at the question raised

The CATS should be limited to 1 page in length. It not only becomes a useful tool for a student or practitioner in the setting of the unique case at hand (whether real or hypothetical), but it also can be archived and used by others with similar case interests or needs. Over time, a wealth of summaries will become available for individual and departmental use. Continuous updating as similar cases and questions arise in the classroom or clinic will ensure that the latest evidence is available. Naming the reviewer permits contact should others want to seek advice, and the date provides a barometer of timeliness so that subsequent users might judge how up-to-date the evidence is.

A template for this learning and teaching activity might look something like that shown in **Table 11.1**, which is my hybridized version of what Sauve et al[3] first described in 1995. Educators, students, and clinicians who find this to be a useful teaching and learning tool should feel free to further adapt it in a manner that best addresses their needs.

Consider Conducting an Evidence-Based Journal Club

There are many approaches to developing a journal club, and no one recipe is best for everyone. What follows are some general guidelines for developing a journal club grounded in the foundations of evidence-based practice. In addition, I have included suggestions that, as a by-product, will subtly instruct attendees in the principles and value of evidence-based practice as a regular component of their professional lives.

Steps for preparing for a journal club meeting include the following:

- Articles, generally targeting a particular theme, are selected by someone with some interest, experience, and expertise in conducting a journal club. In time, a pool of other potential moderators will become available as familiarity with the process is gained.

Table 11.1. Preparing a Critically Appraised Topic Summary (CATS)

Structured template	Example of what to include
Title or area of interest	Postoperative analgesia, drug choice, pediatrics
Focused question (PICO)	How do NSAIDs compare with opiates in relief of pediatric post-tonsillectomy pain, and are there any issues with excessive bleeding?
How was evidence retrieved	Consultation with authoritative providers Journal and book publications cited Electronically accessed databases and sources Other
Describe evidence retrieved	Type of material found and used
Comments about evidence	Brief but critical appraisal of evidence found Description of the primary results
The bottom line	Identification of the clinical take-away point(s)
CATS preparer	Author of this summary
Date of preparation	[insert date]

Abbreviations: PICO, patient, intervention, comparison, outcome; NSAIDs, nonsteroidal anti-inflammatory drugs.

(Modified from Sauve et al.[3])

- It may be beneficial for the coordinator to frame the subject for each journal club meeting with a question posed in the PICO format (see Chapter 2). For example:

  P – In an adult patient undergoing an interscalene block

  I – Does the use of ultrasound-guided needle placement

  C – Compared with electrical stimulation–guided placement

  O – Offer advantages in block quality and rate of complications?

- To avoid overwhelming participants, select 2 to 4 prescreened, high-quality articles, preferably reporting randomized trials or systematic reviews that target the theme.

- Articles should be posted (electronically if possible) about a week in advance for reading.

- It may be helpful to post a few focused questions about the articles under consideration to assist readers in weighing the strength of the evidence. These questions might prompt discussion of the nature of the hypothesis, attributes of the subjects, sample size, methods used, type of analysis undertaken, confounding variables, and major findings.

- Generally, a moderator will assign one person in advance to briefly overview each of the articles.

Recommended steps for conducting an evidence-based journal club meeting are as follows:

- After the assigned person summarizes each article, he or she will open the session for critique and discussion.

- Overall goals of the discussion include the following:
  - Critically appraise the validity and usefulness of the evidence presented
  - Determine the applicability to clinical practice
  - Develop an understanding of the process of evidence-guided patient care
  - Determine how to identify and critique sources of evidence

- It is important to introduce the terms associated with the domain. Randomized control trials, systematic reviews, elements of a good hypothesis, randomization, types of statistical procedures, power, effect size, reliability, validity, and other terms are concepts that may not necessarily be familiar to all participants. Because these terms are encountered in the assigned readings, they should be clarified by the mentor as they arise during the presentation and discussion.

- Each journal club generally concludes with the same general question, "Based on the evidence presented here, would you consider incorporating what has been discussed today into your clinical practice, and if so, under what contextual circumstances?"

- Presentation and discussion should be limited to a finite time (perhaps 30 minutes per article) with a brief break between articles. This limitation helps to keep the meeting interesting and respectful of everyone's time demands.

- Suggestions for topics at future meetings should also be solicited and consideration should be given to evaluating each participant's opinion of the journal club so that future meetings might be improved.

Implementation of an evidence-based journal club is an opportunity to consider practical clinical questions, grounding future interventions more firmly in scientific foundation. Beyond this benefit, it represents the opportunity to engage in the process of EBDM under the tutelage of a mentor who champions the approach. I am a firm believer that the process works best when it helps students and clinicians alike see that an evidence-based process is highly relevant to everyday anesthetic practice and is achievable. Journal club meetings should be focused on questions that are highly relevant to clinical practice. Use of the PICO approach (see Chapter 2) will help everyone formulate high-quality, clinically based questions and will provide the mentor or teacher with an opportunity to reveal the benefits of endeavoring to use evidence in future practice.

References

1. Combs AW. Fostering maximum development of the individual. In: van Til W, Rehage KJ, eds. *Issues in Secondary Education.* (NSSE Yearbook, 1976, Vol 74, Issue 2). Chicago, IL: National Society for the Study of Education; 1976.

2. Marzano RJ. *A Different Kind of Classroom: Teaching With Dimensions of Learning.* Alexandria, VA: Association for Supervision and Curriculum Development; 1992.

3. Sauve S, Lee HN, Meade MO, et al. The critically appraised topic: a practical approach to learning critical appraisal. *Ann Roy Coll Physicians Surg Canada.* 1995;28:396-398.

CHAPTER TWELVE

A Crash Course in Common Statistical Tests for the Nonstatistician

Many of us may lack confidence in our understanding of statistical analysis. At some level, however, we recognize that statistics are essential not only to the research process itself but also to engaging in an evidence-based approach to patient care. This chapter is a brief overview for the nonstatistician of some of the common statistical procedures encountered in the biomedical literature. But before we get started, a little story:

> A man set out in a hot-air balloon and soon found himself lost, with little in the way of landmarks except for fields of grass as far as he could see. Eventually, he saw a man directly beneath him who was walking his dog. Leaning over the basket he yelled out, "Hello sir! Where am I?"
>
> The man walking the dog looked up and replied, "You're about 30 feet above the ground in a hot-air balloon."
>
> The balloonist, quite frustrated, shouted back, "You must be a statistician."
>
> "Indeed I am! How could you possibly know that?" asked the man on the ground.
>
> "Well," retorted the balloonist, "You're absolutely correct, but your answer was completely useless."
>
> "I see," replied the walker, "And you sir, must be a manager."
>
> "In fact, you're quite right," said the balloonist. "How on earth did you know?"
>
> "Well," said the walker, "first you were lost. Then, trying to work out what information you needed to sort yourself out, you asked someone else to get it for you. Now that you have the information, you're still lost, but it's someone else's fault."

In our careers as nurse anesthetists, we are charged with making complex decisions that have short-term and long-term consequences for patients. These decisions are often predicated on understanding and using statistics, which, despite the criticism leveled by the balloonist, actually have an essential purpose—to facilitate understanding and use of information in clinical practice.

When I think of statistical analysis, I consider what this family of tools can do for me, such as the following:

- Provide a summary of numeric information in a concise manner.
- Assist me to understand and test a hypothesis—for example, mobile phones cause brain tumors—and, in that process, give me an indication of how certain the conclusion is.
- Help me compare information from different groups—for example, how does the outcome of patients receiving intervention X compare with that of patients receiving intervention Y?
- Facilitate predictions of just how likely an event is for a particular patient—for example, when will I need to redose an epidural or redose a muscle relaxant—and provide an estimate of how accurate the prediction is.

Descriptive statistical procedures simply summarize important quantitative information about a population or a sample of a population. Common descriptive statistics include such things as height, weight, gender, ASA classification, comorbidity, and selected physiologic variables. Often, these statistics are presented as a range of values (low to high), a frequency, or a mean. *Inferential statistical procedures* are designed to allow us to make inferences beyond our particular sampled population. For example, we collect data on a representative sample of subjects from a population and, on that basis, make estimations (or conjectures) about the larger population. Along the way, there are many important questions to consider so that final inferences are valid (**Figure 12.1**).

Parametric and Nonparametric Tests

Information can be presented in many forms. Data measured on a numeric, low to high scale are referred to as *continuous* or *interval*. Measurements such as temperature, heart rate, amount of blood loss, and end-tidal agent concentration are examples. *Discrete* or *ordinal* data have some sort of rank order, but the scale may not be linear. For example, on a visual analog scale in which "0" represents no pain and "10" denotes the worst pain imaginable, a score of "8" for pain does not necessarily mean that pain is twice as intense as pain represented by a score of "4." *Dichotomous* or *binary* data are simply "yes/no" or "absent/present" in nature, such as whether a patient is alive or dead after a defined study period or whether a patient is intubated or not intubated before transfer from the operating room. *Categorical* or *nominal* data suggest different groupings but do not involve any kind of rank ordering; placing different patients in categories of different preoperative comorbidities is an example. The test chosen to analyze the data is based on the key properties of the data and the nature of the research question or hypothesis under consideration. **Table 12.1** summarizes the uses of some commonly used statistical procedures.

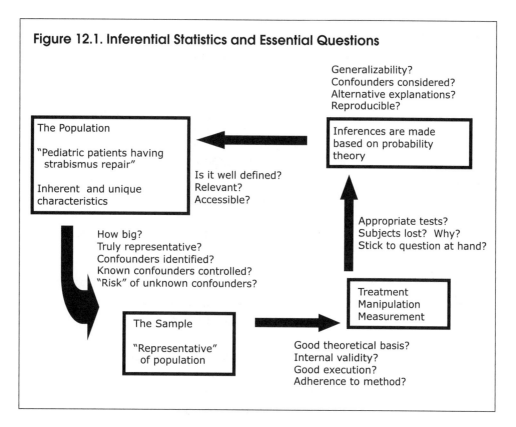

Figure 12.1. Inferential Statistics and Essential Questions

Parametric Tests

Parametric tests are more robust and, for the most part, require fewer data to make a stronger conclusion than nonparametric tests. However, to use a parametric test, a few assumptions must be met. These assumptions include the following: (1) The data need to be normally distributed, that is, they must follow a bell-shaped curve when displayed on a histogram-type plot. (2) The data need to have equal variance and the same standard deviation. (3) The data need to be continuous (on a numeric scale from low to high). Parametric tests frequently encountered in the literature are briefly described in this section.

The assumption of data being normally distributed is based in part on what is known as the *central limit theorem of statistics*. This complex sounding phrase simply states that the sum of a sufficiently large number of independent random variables approaches a normal distribution, whether it be height, weight, heart rate, blood volume, IQ, speed in a 1-mile race, or hematocrit concentration. Much of the data acquired in healthcare as well as economics, baseball, and the transportation industry are obtained in the aggregate—adding up all obtained measures over some time period. In as much as each unique measure occurs independently and even randomly, we would, over time and in the aggregate, expect the variations in the total data pool to be approximately normal in their distribution.

Table 12.1. Commonly Used Statistical Procedures: Selecting the Right Statistical Test Based on Data Type and Purpose

Use this test category	If the data are of this type
Parametric	Interval or ratio (numeric scale, the data distribution is "normal," ie, in a bell shape). Also, the samples that are compared have similar variance, and observations in a group are independent.
Nonparametric	Nominal or ordinal, or assumptions for the parametric tests are not met.
	Data are considered "distribution free"; good for small samples in which observations in a group are independent.

Use this test	If the goal is
Analysis of variance	Test the difference among the means of 2 or more independent groups or more than 1 independent variable.
Analysis of covariance	Test for differences between group means after adjustment of the scores on the dependent variable to eliminate the effects of a covariate.
Chi-square test (χ^2)	Evaluate the difference between observed and expected frequencies.
Correlation coefficient	Test whether a relationship or association exists between 2 variables.
Pearson	Dependent and independent variables are continuous (interval).
Spearman	Calculate a correlation between ordinal-level data.
Factor analysis	Reduce a large set of variables into a more manageable set of measures.
Kaplan-Meier curve	Probability of surviving, or not surviving, a particular event over time.
Kruskal-Wallis test	Similar to a 1-way analysis of variance but using ordinal data; it is an extension of the Mann-Whitney test for 3 or more groups.
Mann-Whitney (U) test	Compare 2 groups that have ordinal-level data.
Multiple linear regression	Understand the effects of 2 or more independent variables on a dependent measure.

Table continues on page 119.

Use this test	If the goal is
Simple linear regression	Use 1 independent variable *(x)* to predict a dependent variable *(y)*.
t Test, independent groups	Test the difference between the means of 2 independent groups.
t Test, dependent samples	Test for the difference between dependent, paired samples (eg, pretreatment and posttreatment outcome).
Wilcoxon rank sum test	Compare 2 groups that have ordinal-level data (see Mann-Whitney *(U)* test).
Wilcoxon signed ranks test	Use as alternative to *t* test when a normal distribution of the data cannot be assumed.

Pearson Product Moment Correlation

The correlation coefficient (r) indicates just how well 2 continuous-scaled variables from the same subject or subject group are associated with one another. When $r = 1.0$, the variables are perfectly positively correlated. When $r = 0$, there is an absolutely random or meaningless correlation. When $r = -1.0$, there is a perfectly negative correlation. Values between these limits demonstrate intermediate correlations (**Figure 12.2**).

Other correlation coefficients are available besides the Pearson product moment correlation. To determine associations between variables that are not both continuous-scaled measures, for example, a case in which both variables are of rank order, the Kendall tau (τ) can be used. When one variable is dichotomous (binary) and the other variable is on a continuous scale, the point-biserial correlational technique can be used. When both variables are dichotomous, the phi (φ) coefficient technique can be used. The Spearman coefficient is also in the family of correlational procedures and will be described separately in the section "Nonparametric Tests."

Another correlation computation sometimes encountered in the biomedical literature, the coefficient of determination (r^2), is an estimate of how much a change in one variable influences the other. For example, in a study of core temperature and oxygen consumption, $r = 0.9$ (a very powerful, positive correlation, as might be expected). The calculated r^2, $(0.9^2) = 0.81$, suggests that 81% of the variability in oxygen consumption is explained by the patient's core temperature.

A caution should be mentioned. Commonly, nurse anesthetists want to learn about how 2 different measures of a phenomenon compare (eg, invasive vs noninvasive cardiac output or determining oxygen consumption with inspired gas analysis vs the reverse Fick method) to determine if the methods agree sufficiently to be used interchangeably. Correlation is simply a measure of association, although it is often improperly used to

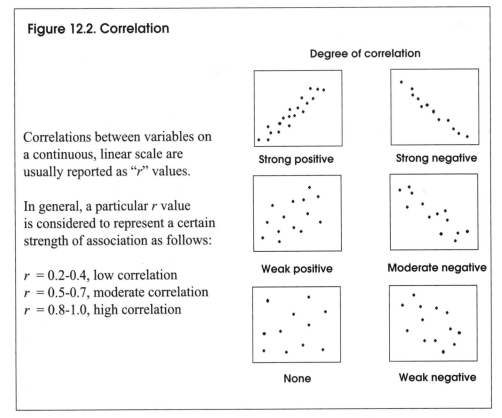

Figure 12.2. Correlation

Degree of correlation

Correlations between variables on a continuous, linear scale are usually reported as "*r*" values.

In general, a particular *r* value is considered to represent a certain strength of association as follows:

r = 0.2-0.4, low correlation
r = 0.5-0.7, moderate correlation
r = 0.8-1.0, high correlation

Strong positive

Strong negative

Weak positive

Moderate negative

None

Weak negative

determine agreement. In this case, the *Bland-Altman plot* is the more appropriate tool to use. This tool initially determines the difference in measured values in the same subject. The mean of the differences in a sample of subjects is the estimated bias (ie, the difference between the methods), and the standard deviation of the differences measures the random variability around this mean value. Limits of agreements are established (usually 1 or 2 SDs) between the methods, and if these agreement boundaries are met, the conclusion is often that the 2 methods are interchangeable.

In addition, a kappa statistic (κ) is frequently seen in the scientific literature. It is used to quantify the agreement between 2 raters who are determining a variable or outcome on a categorical scale. A κ of 1.0 suggests perfect agreement, and a κ of 0 suggests no agreement other than what might occur by chance alone. Different texts vary slightly in their interpretation of the κ value, but, in general, a computed value of 0.6 to 1.0 is considered very strong, values less than 0.3 are considered weak, and values between 0.3 and 0.6 are considered moderate.

Regression Analysis

Although correlation provides information about the degree of association, regression analysis assists in making predictions about how a change in one variable affects another variable. Examples include the effect of patient age on inhalational drug requirement, the plasma concentration of a drug and its attendant pharmacodynamics, and the effects of a given cardiac output on renal blood flow. In plots of such relationships, the *dependent variable* (the outcome) conventionally is placed on the y-axis and the *independent variable* (the manipulated variable or the predictor variable), on the x-axis.

A 19th century scientist, Sir Francis Galton (who, by the way, also introduced us to the concept of the sleeping bag), was a Renaissance man in the truest sense of the term. His scientific interest was in the domain of determining mathematical methods to assess and predict human measurements. A classic example of his work involved predicting the physical attributes of children, such as height, based on the attributes of the parents. Galton's pioneering work laid the foundation for subsequent use of regression analysis as a predictive mathematical tool.

In plotting relationship for this analytical procedure, the researcher can calculate a "line of best fit" or the "regression" line by using a procedure known as the "method of least squares." With the use of this technique, regression analysis provides a way to describe, interpret, and predict the relationship between 2 variables measured on a continuous scale.

As with other statistical procedures, the accuracy of any procedure in describing a relationship is likely to be imperfect. This imperfection (or uncertainty) can be quantified in terms of the *standard error* and the *confidence interval,* or CI. In general, these measures of uncertainty shrink somewhat as the sample size increases—greater amounts of sampling generally improve "certainty" about what is going on. The CI is often expressed as a 95% CI. I think of this as meaning that 19 times of 20 (ie, 95%), the "true value" sampled in a population will be in the specified range of values.

Because the CI is so widely used in published reports, some elaboration might prove illuminating. I think of the CI as the range in which the true treatment effect is likely to lie. The CI is, in general, preferable to *P*-values in that it better aids interpretation of trial data by putting an upper and lower boundary on the likely effect size of any real effect. Additionally if the CI includes the value of no difference (ie, the value "1.0") then there is no significant difference from the reference group. Finally, statistical significance does not necessarily mean clinical significance (and vice versa). Any reported finding must be put in the context of the study population and great care must be exercised in applying any research findings to a particular patient.

Regression analysis provides tools that allow assessment of the relationship between 1 dependent (outcome) variable and 1 or more independent (manipulated or predictor) variables. *Multiple regression* is yet another approach in which 2 or more independent variables are combined to predict a dependent variable. *Stepwise regression* analysis is commonly used in anesthesia research because it provides the ability to weigh the impact of a number of independent variables separately or in combination to determine or predict their effect on an outcome. For example, in a study of atelectasis formation during general anesthesia, select variables such as body habitus, surgery type, surgery duration, smoking history, gender, comorbidity, and anesthesia management would be considered by both their independent and combined effects on atelectasis formation. Stepwise regression would be ideally suited to this task.

Because *linear regression* analysis is so widely used in biomedical research, I am going to offer some key points to improve understanding of its role:

- Linear regression is used when a strong and significant correlation between 2 variables is demonstrated, allowing you to make predictions about 1 variable based on your appreciation for the other.
- The more powerful the correlation coefficient is, the greater the likelihood that the regression model will hold true.
- Linear regression works only when there is an established linear relationship between the variables under consideration.
- When fitting linear models, our hope is to find that 1 variable (Y, heart rate) is varying in a relatively straight-line function of another variable (X, dose of a β-blocker).
- The final computed regression line is a kind of moving average that summarizes the balancing point of observations made at each point on the x-axis.
- The concepts of *homoscedasticity* and *heteroscedasticity* are important in linear regression applications. The former indicates that the variability in scores for the independent variable is the same for all values of the dependent variable; with the latter, that relationship is not consistent.

Figure 12.3 illustrates the utility of linear regression.

Student *t* Test

Statistical tests are designed to accept or reject the assumed null hypothesis (ie, there are no differences between groups). The *t* test is probably the most common parametric test encountered. Three types of Student *t* test are used to test the null hypothesis that there is no difference between 2 group means. A 1-sample *t* test is used to determine whether the mean of a sample is different from the mean of a known, at-large population. An unpaired *t* test is used when 2 independent samples are compared, such as comparing the effect on blood pressure of 2 different manipulations performed during laryngoscopy. A paired *t* test is used on 2 dependent samples, such as might occur when preintervention and postintervention group scores are compared in the same group of subjects.

The *t*-test calculation uses the mean, standard deviation, and number of samples to calculate the test statistic. For reasons that are not fully clear, the traditional level of significance is a *P* value of less than .05 (see the discussion on this point in Chapter 5) so that in a data set with a relatively large number of samples, the critical value for the *t* test is 1.96 for an α (*P* value) of .05, obtained from a *t*-test table. The calculation to determine the *t* value can be found easily online or in the most elementary statistics

Figure 12.3. Linear Regression

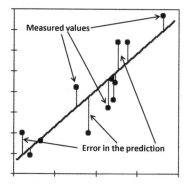

Measured values

Error in the prediction

The regression line minimizes the sum of the squared vertical distances between actual data measurements made. It is the "line of best fit."

In virtually any prediction there is bound to be some error. Although prediction will not be perfect, regression permits a systematic and rational approach that vastly improves merely guessing or relying on intuition!

The *straight-line formula* is used to predict the value of *Y* for any given value of *X* (or vice versa). Predictions should be made only within the range of observed values; going beyond leads to extrapolation that can yield false results.

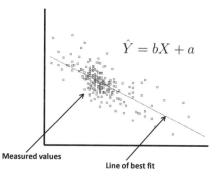

$$\hat{Y} = bX + a$$

Measured values

Line of best fit

Homoscedasticity **Heteroscedasticity**

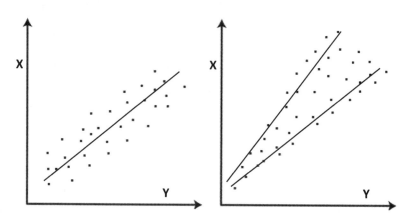

Scatter plot at bottom left reveals the residuals as approximately equal for all predicted values. Think this way: the variability in one random score at one point is approximately the same as that seen in another random score at another point on the line. Scatter plot at bottom right reveals an approximate linear relationship between *X* and *Y*, but more importantly, it reveals a statistical condition termed *heteroscedasticity* (ie, "different variation"). Here the vertical variation in *Y* differs depending on the value of *X*. In this example, small values of *X* yield small scatter in *Y* while large values of *X* result in large scatter in Y.

books. The P value is essentially the risk of making a type I error—the risk of falsely rejecting the null hypothesis—in other words, claiming a difference between groups when one does not exist. The t test should not be used for comparisons involving more than 2 groups.

The z Test

The z-test statistic is calculated for samples that are relatively large where the data do not have to reflect a normal distribution. It is used most often to determine the percentage of the standard population's test scores that are outside the mean of the sample population. Traditionally, as with the t test, if more than 95% of the standard population is on one side of the mean, the P value is less than .05 and statistical significance is achieved.

Analysis of Variance

The analysis of variance (ANOVA) is another very common parametric test, one that incorporates group means and variances to determine the test statistic. The test statistic is then used to determine whether 2 or more groups of data vary from one another in a meaningful way. As with other statistical procedures, the ANOVA assumes that the null hypothesis is stated such that all group means are the same. The ANOVA then accepts or rejects the null hypothesis. The test statistic for ANOVA is called the F ratio.

The ANOVA can be used to compare 2 group means in the same manner as the t test. The decision to accept or reject the null hypothesis is based on the preestablished α (P value), that is, the chance of making a type I error (see Table 5.2).

When comparing the means of 3 or more groups, the ANOVA is referred to as a 1-way or 1-factor ANOVA. Other forms of ANOVA include the 2-way ANOVA, when 2 different grouping factors are used, and the multiple ANOVA (sometimes called MANOVA), when multiple grouping factors are analyzed. The ANOVA with repeated-measures test is commonly used; as with the standard ANOVA, it tests the equality of means. When all members of a random sample's dependent variable are measured under a number of different conditions or repeatedly measured over time, the ANOVA with repeated measures is used.

Should the ANOVA indicate that a significant difference exists when more than 2 groups are compared, it cannot localize where the groups differ, only that there is a difference somewhere. In this case, a *post hoc test* must be used to isolate the between- or among-group difference. There are many of these tests, and different computer programs and statisticians have their favorites; examples include the Fisher, Scheffé, Tukey, Newman-Keuls, and Dunnett tests.

Nonparametric Tests

Data failing to meet the criteria for a parametric test are analyzed with a nonparametric instrument. Generally speaking, nonparametric tests require more data (eg, larger sample or more measurement points) to reach a valid conclusion. Because the data sets that are amenable to nonparametric procedures are not normally distributed, they are sometimes referred to as distribution-free tests.

Chi-Square

The chi-square (χ^2) test is a commonly used tool for comparing groups of categorical or frequency data. It determines the extent that a single observed set of measures differs from a theoretical or expected set of measures. It is useful in addressing the question, What is the extent that an observed distribution deviates from a theoretical or expected distribution? The data categories must be mutually exclusive and discrete, and only actual counts (frequencies) can be used in the calculation.

Along the same lines as the χ^2 test is the Fisher exact test. This test is used if the cell counts (a cell constitutes a unique value at the intersection of a treatment and an outcome in the table) are particularly small (usually < 5). Because of its complexity, it necessitates a computer program to calculate, although some mathematical aficionados might dismiss this assertion.

Spearman Rank Coefficient

The Spearman rank coefficient, also known as the Spearman rho (ρ) coefficient, is used to estimate the strength and direction of association between 2 ordinal variables. Like the Pearson product moment correlation, its calculated value ranges from -1.00 to 1.00. A positive coefficient indicates that the value of one variable varies in the same direction as another variable. A negative coefficient indicates that the values vary in opposite directions.

For example, in a study that seeks to identify the relationship of patients' ASA classifications with the type of airway management that the patients receive, the authors of the study might rank the airway interventions by "degree of invasiveness," such as tracheostomy > endotracheal intubation > laryngeal mask airway > face mask > natural (none). Given that both variables are ordinal, the ρ coefficient would provide one approach to describing the nature of their association.

Mann-Whitney Test

The Mann-Whitney test is also referred to as the U test or the Wilcoxon rank sum test. Analogous to the t test for continuous variables, this test compares 2 independent populations for some ordinal measure to determine whether they are different. The sample values from both sets of data are ranked together. Once test statistics are calculated, the individual groups are compared with one another to determine if a significant difference exists. This test is commonly used when there are more than 2 categories (eg, "excellent, reasonable, and poor") that in some way rank attributes associated with them.

For example, in a study of postoperative analgesia in the first 24 hours following bilateral inguinal hernia repair in 40 men randomly assigned to receive codeine and acetaminophen or ibuprofen and acetaminophen, the subjects rate their pain scores 16 hours postoperatively. All of the pain scores are recorded and ranked from lowest to highest. The test then determines whether the sum of the ranks in one group (eg, the codeine and acetaminophen group) differs from the sum of the ranks in the other group (eg, the ibuprofen and acetaminophen group).

Kruskal-Wallis Test

The Kruskal-Wallis test can be viewed as the nonparametric alternative to a 1-way ANOVA. The Kruskal-Wallis test does not make assumptions about normal distribution and is performed on data that are ranked in some manner; the observations measured in the original data collection are transformed so that the smallest value is ranked "1.0," the next smallest is ranked "2.0," and so forth.

The Kruskal-Wallis test is ideally suited for comparing 3 or more groups in which all of the data are ranked numerically and the rank values are then summed and averaged for each group. If the null hypothesis that all groups are drawn from the same population is true, the mean ranks should be similar across all groups. If a significant difference among the groups is encountered, a post hoc test is usually performed to isolate exactly which groups differ from one another.

Power Analysis

Performing power analysis and sample size estimation is an essential step in planning and executing an experimental design. *Power* refers to the ability of a statistical test to detect a significant effect if, in fact, one exists. Failure to do this calculation may lead to researchers engaging in research interventions in which the sample size (n) may be too high or too low. If the n is too low, the experiment will lack the ability to provide reliable answers to the questions it is investigating. If the n is too large, time and resources may be unnecessarily wasted, often for minimal gain. A more thorough discussion of power analysis and sample size calculation is provided in Chapter 13, "A Practical Guide for Achieving Statistical Power: Just How Much Is Enough?"

The Rule of Three: What's That?

In prelicensure clinical trials, adverse event detection is crucially important but when such events are very rare, detection often does not occur until postmarketing surveillance reveals them. One approach that is commonly used in this and other settings of rare adverse events is the so-called "rule of three."

The rule is based on the estimated upper limit of the 95% confidence interval when a particular adverse event has not occurred. It is succinctly stated as, if no major adverse events have occurred in a group sized as N, there is a 95% confidence that the chance of major adverse events is less than 1 in N/3. Although the theoretical underpinnings will not be detailed here, most argue that the application of this rule works best when N > 30.

As an example, assume that we are evaluating a newly released local anesthetic that remarkably has not been associated with any immunologic, cardiovascular, or neurogenic adverse reactions in the reported trial involving 1,500 surgical patients. The "rule of three" suggests that we should have 95% confidence that the rate of adverse events is not going to exceed 1 in 500 patients in whom we used the drug. Here is another example. Ever driven your car and wondered if the airbag housed in your steering wheel would actually deploy if needed? Let's assume that a car manufacturer, "Reliable

Wheels," has randomly tested 300 cars by deliberately crashing them head-on into a foam-covered brick wall. In each crash the airbag deployed successfully. Using the "rule of three" we can conclude, with 95% confidence, that the chance of an airbag failing in another group of 300 would be 3/N (ie, 3/300) or 1 in 100.

Displaying Time-to-Event Data: Kaplan-Meier Curve

The use of the Kaplan-Meier survival analysis is increasingly seen in the anesthesia literature and has great utility for displaying the time course of an outcome of some nature. The types of outcomes for which this is useful include the time it takes to report relief of pain or nausea, time to onset of a surgical site infection, time for a "cure" to be reached, or time to reach a catastrophic outcome such as myocardial infarction, stroke or even death. The Kaplan-Meier curve descriptively displays an outcome when time to that outcome is the important variable. **Figure 12.4** illustrates the use of Kaplan-Meier analysis in a study examining the relationship over time of intraoperative hypotension on all-cause mortality.

Although Kaplan-Meier analysis has great application to clarifying the time until a subject presents with a defined outcome, it also has great utility in the exploratory stages of a study when relationships are in the early stages of being assessed.

Some Brief Thoughts About Recursive Partitioning

Recursive partitioning is a commonly used tool that is based on a rule set that allows for decision making using a set of questions vs using equations. The term *recursive* pertains to using a rule or procedure that can be applied repeatedly, and *partitioning* refers to the subsequent division (or partitioning) into portions or shares.

The process usually involves nonparametric data (binary or dichotomous), multiple variables, and a decision tree with a rule such as "if a patient has findings *x, y, and z* then the patient probably has *q*." This can help predict a number of things such as risk, mortality, and best treatment approach. The Goldman cardiac risk stratification, where accumulated points for different pathophysiological attributes indicate the potential for mortality, or the STOP-Bang inventory, used commonly in preanesthetic assessment of the patient for risk of obstructive sleep apnea, are examples of processes based on recursive partitioning.

Figure 12.5 illustrates a potential use of recursive partitioning in arriving at a decision, using the metaphor of an upside-down tree, and provides a common tool (ASA Difficult Airway Algorithm) as an example.

Recursive partitioning generates useful clinical information without the burden of doing mathematical calculations, providing a fairly simple map to help negotiate cognitive processes that may involve many complex variables. The major drawbacks to its application is that it is not well suited to parametric (continuous)–type variables and also that a mistake made early in the decision-making tree can lead one astray, providing incorrect directionality and analysis.

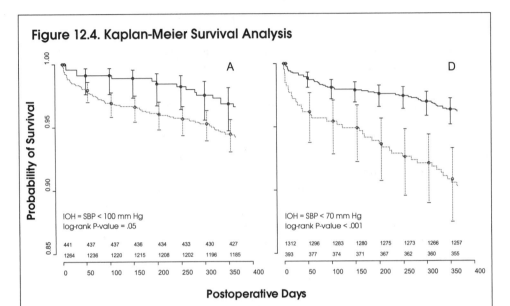

Figure 12.4. Kaplan-Meier Survival Analysis

Analysis of death due to all causes in relationship to intraoperative hypotension (IOH). Panel **A** graphs all-cause mortality in those patients who had a systolic blood pressure (SBP) continuously >100 mm Hg (solid line) compared with those who had a SBP < 100 mm Hg for at least 1 minute (broken line). Panel **D** graphs all-cause mortality in those patients who had a SBP continuously > 100 mm Hg compared with those who had a SBP < 70 mm Hg for at least 1 minute. Although not proposing a cause-and-effect relationship, the authors concluded that mortality increased when the degree of IOH increased, indicating the relationship requires further study.

Vertical bars represent the 95% CIs at each 50-day increment. Above the x-axis upper row of numbers indicates the upper curve; lower row, lower curve.

(Adapted from Bijker JB, van Klei WA, Vergouwe Y et al. Intraoperative hypotension and 1-year mortality after noncardiac surgery. *Anesthesiology.* 2009;111(6):1217-1226.)

Summary

This review of some of the common statistical tests encountered in clinical research literature is not meant to be comprehensive or prescriptive. Just as there are many variations in the way that anesthesia is conducted, even variation in how a single drug is administered, approaches to data analysis using conventional statistical tools are subject to great variability. To practice evidence-based anesthesia, nurse anesthetists do not need to be experts at understanding statistics or be able to perform the tests themselves. What is desired is to have an understanding of what tests are generally appropriate for a given data type and whether a particular test is appropriate to illuminate the hypothesis at hand. Understanding the fundamental use of these tests should provide a framework for critiquing and better understanding published reports of clinical research, thus enhancing nurse anesthetists' ability for evidence-based practice.

Figure 12.5. Recursive Partitioning

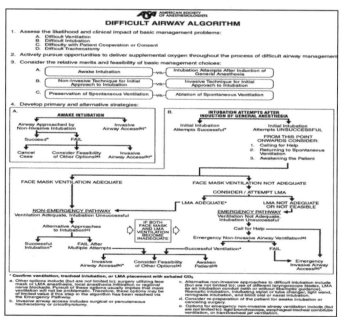

In the top illustration, moving from the "trunk" of the tree to the leaves through a series of "yes/no" questions leads to greater and finer discrimination. Considering the trunk as the common population and each leaf as an individual, with repeated questioning, isolation of a particular leaf or group of leaves becomes possible. Recursive partitioning is the fundamental process employed in the ASA "Difficult Airway Algorithm" (at bottom), providing us with the best option or options in a particular setting by advancing through the matrix using dichotomous (yes/no) questions.

CHAPTER THIRTEEN

A Practical Guide for Achieving Statistical Power: Just How Much Is Enough?

esearch works best when it is thoughtfully planned and executed according to that plan. There are many components to a good plan, for example, attention to suitable subject selection, use of valid and reliable instruments, unambiguous operationalization of terms, and appropriate attention to "sizing" the study sample relative to the investigator's goals. It is this latter consideration that will be discussed here, for as we shall see it's not just about it being big enough, as being too big can create problems just as concerning.

We can begin by considering why sample size is so important when planning or evaluating a study. The first thing that comes to mind is the matter of cost of the study. An *undersized* study may not have the capacity to meet the investigator's goals, wasting time and resources in the process. If the study is underpowered, it may unnecessarily expose subjects to an intervention or exposure that might be risky or even harmful, not meeting an important ethical threshold. Likewise, an underpowered study simply fails to advance knowledge and in the worst-case scenario provides incorrect information.

In the case of the *oversized* study too many subjects may be placed at potential harm (dependent on the nature of the intervention) due to exposure to a new intervention. In a randomized trial, subjects may be denied what has been traditionally viewed as a beneficial intervention (if assigned to the control or common treatment group). Oversized studies may be unnecessarily expensive, consuming time, resources, and talent beyond what is required. An additional hazard is that if the sample size is too large, the results may provide a false statistical inference.

What Is Statistical Power?

You should broadly think of statistical power, or a power analysis, to be the probability of actually detecting statistically significant differences between (or among) the data groups in a study if, in fact, such differences exist (**Figure 13.1**). In statistical parlance, power is viewed as the probability of rejecting a false null hypothesis. Typically, a study's power is set at 0.80, which implies that there is an 80% chance of finding differences that truly exist. Although that value may not sound very high (wouldn't 90% or 95% or 100% be better?), it is a reasonable value given the logistics of doing research and has become traditional over

Figure 13.1. Does the Study Have Enough "Octane" (Power) to Address the Hypothesis?

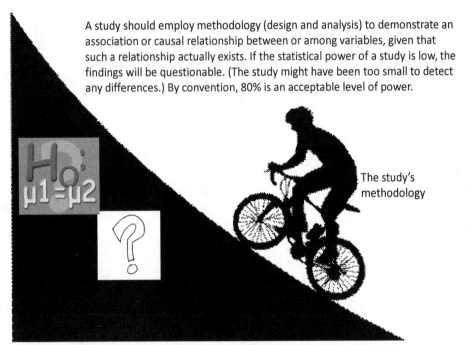

A study should employ methodology (design and analysis) to demonstrate an association or causal relationship between or among variables, given that such a relationship actually exists. If the statistical power of a study is low, the findings will be questionable. (The study might have been too small to detect any differences.) By convention, 80% is an acceptable level of power.

The study's methodology

Demonstrating that the cyclist (representing the study methods) has the power to actually get up the hill (the challenge of addressing the null hypothesis) should be determined and reported in the write-up of the study.

the decades. How statisticians and researchers 100 years from now will view this is up for conjecture! **Table 13.1** is a summary of the major statistical power issues.

For those readers who are interested in how the "80% chance" became traditional, see the nota bene at the end of this chapter. I will spare the less-interested reader here from these details.

How Can Statistical Power Be Amplified?

There are 2 kinds of sample sizes that should be computed in an ideal world. The first is a determination of how many subjects need to be recruited to actually be representative of the population at large. A second determination is directed at the issue noted earlier—importing enough "octane" or "horsepower" to your study to allow you reject a false null hypothesis.

Table 13.1. Summary of Statistical Power Issues

- Statistical power $(1 - \beta)$ is the probability of rejecting a false null hypothesis.
- Statistical power is wedded to type I error (P, α) and type II error (β).
- Sample size, effect size, and directionality of the hypothesis influence statistical power.
- Effect size is not controlled by the researcher; the other factors are modifiable.
- The largest single factor influencing statistical power is the sample size.
- Carefully consider the issue of statistical power when you fail to reject the null hypothesis.
- Whether as a clinician-reader or a researcher, carefully consider the power issue.

The major ways of increasing power are the following:

- Increasing the sample size
- Increasing the "alpha" (α) level
- Using a 1-tailed test (ie, using a directional, < or > statement of the hypothesis)
- Employing highly valid and reliable measures in the study
- Preparing a very strong research design (methodology)

The statistical procedure that the researcher uses greatly influences the ultimate sample size calculation. For example, the calculation of an appropriate sample size is different for a correlation analysis than it is for analysis of variance. Likewise, the effect size plays prominently in sample size or power considerations (**Figure 13.2**).

Sample Size and Effect Size

The *effect size* is the magnitude of the relationship between the independent variable (the manipulated variable, or variable of interest) and the dependent variable (the outcome of interest). Effect sizes are reported as small, medium, or large. Think of this example:

> The time to "street fitness" following a single intravenous dose of 2 mg/kg of propofol for anesthetic induction
>
> compared with
>
> Time to street fitness after a single dose of 0.2 mg/kg of midazolam for anesthetic induction

In this example the effect size (the expected impact of the drug on the outcome) would be expected to be very large.

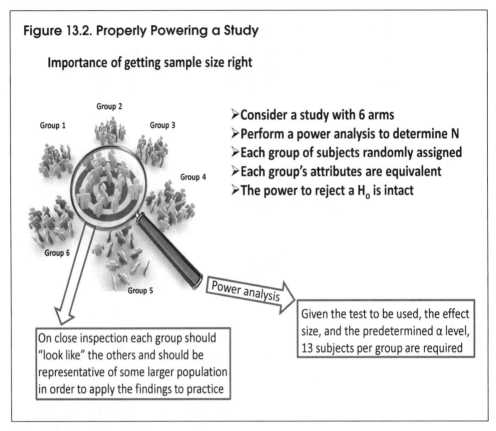

Figure 13.2. Properly Powering a Study

Importance of getting sample size right

➤Consider a study with 6 arms
➤Perform a power analysis to determine N
➤Each group of subjects randomly assigned
➤Each group's attributes are equivalent
➤The power to reject a H_0 is intact

Power analysis

On close inspection each group should "look like" the others and should be representative of some larger population in order to apply the findings to practice

Given the test to be used, the effect size, and the predetermined α level, 13 subjects per group are required

Abbreviation: H_0, null hypothesis.

Now consider this example:

> Mortality in healthy male patients undergoing general anesthesia for inguinal hernia repair with sevoflurane

> compared with

> Mortality in health male patients undergoing general anesthesia for inguinal hernia repair with isoflurane

In this example the effect size (the expected impact of the drug on the outcome) would be expected to be small.

Because effect size strongly influences the ability to detect differences in the comparison groups, a large, readily detectable effect (as in the propofol vs midazolam example) would require a relatively small sample size to demonstrate group differences. However, in the case of a very small effect size (as in the sevoflurane vs isoflurane example) an enormously large sample size would be needed, even if an effect were actually present—in this case unlikely! **Table 13.2** reviews the important elements affecting power.

The ideal time to calculate power is before the study has occurred (termed an a *priori analysis*), thus providing a theoretical foundation for how many subjects should be studied. Knowledge of the 3 factors noted in Table 13.2 allows us to calculate a fourth, beta (β). Looking back at Table 5.2, we see that α is the probability of a type I error (rejection of a true null hypothesis), whereas β is the probability of a type II error (acceptance of a false null hypothesis).

Performing a Power Analysis

Using programs accessible on the Internet (many of which are free), a researcher can perform a power analysis (or you can redo an analysis that has already been done!) in the following way. Here is a study I created (as a thought experiment only) to illustrate the process:

Using a standard apparatus checkout procedure for drug and equipment setup for the first case of the day, we find that an average of 11 minutes is required by a provider. I wish to perform a study using a voice recording to prompt the provider to accomplish these tasks, and I hypothesize that the voice prompting will decrease the time required to perform the collective of tasks. I suggest that the effect size is moderate based on my review of the literature and that a 3-minute decrease in that time would represent a reasonable and practically important improvement. I also plan to have the same number of individuals in my control group (the standard procedure without the voice prompt) and the experimental group (the recorded voice prompt group).

In conducting a power analysis, I went to one of the many programs on the Internet and input the requested values. I selected "sample size for comparing means of two independent groups" from a large menu of choices. The groups in my study are independent, and the data recorded (minutes) represent the kind of data amenable to a *t* test (ie, bell-shaped distribution with reasonable variance).

Table 13.2. Summary of Factors That Affect Power

Factor	Definition
Alpha (α)	Traditionally set at .05. It is the probability of believing we have found a difference when one is not there.
Sample size (N)	In general, a larger sample size provides us with a more precise estimate of a parameter. Here the more intense and wider the search, the more likely we may find it.
Effect size	Magnitude of the phenomenon that occurs in the population. Think of it this way: the larger it is, the more readily it will be detected.

Sample size for comparing means of 2 independent groups (unpaired t test)

How: Enter the number of groups, the anticipated within-group standard deviation, and the anticipated differences or the minimal difference that is of interest in the appropriate text boxes. Click Calculate button, and the results will show.

| .3 | Anticipated difference in means   [Calculate]

| 0.5 | Anticipated effect size (small = 0.2, moderate = 0.5, large = 0.8)

| 1 | Ratio of control to experimental subjects

Sample size estimates per group for independent groups (unpaired t test)

Assuming that all observations are independent:

	Type I error = .05	**Type I error = .01**	**Type I error = .001**
Power = 80%	45	67	98
Power = 90%	60	85	119
Power = 99%	104	136	178

Interpretation: Here we see the program provides us with sample size calculations based on what α and β values we elect to use. In this a priori analysis, to conduct a study with an α = .05 and a β = 80%, we would require 64 cases per group. You can see that increasing the demands on α or β will lead to an increased need for subjects in each group.

Is Bigger Always Better?

It is important to adequately size a study, and this responsibility, while falling on the investigator and later the publishing journal's editors, ultimately defaults to the readers of the study report as they judge the merit and clinical applicability of the investigator's work. A study needs to be large enough so that the methodology employed can detect group differences if, in fact, such differences exist. So why not just use very large sample sizes in all studies?

It is equally important that a study not employ an excessively large sample size. In such cases an effect of little scientific or clinical relevance might arise. Likewise, there are compelling economic and resource implications for a study that is too large. Although an undersized study can erode time, talent, and other resources for not having the "octane" to produce useful outcomes, an oversized study will consume more resources (time, talent, money) than is necessary. In addition, an oversized study may actually create ethical issues in the face of potentially hazardous interventions (ie, manipulations with an adverse event profile). The bottom line for the statistically and mathematically oriented reader is this: when the sample size is too large, hypothesis testing becomes biased in favor of rejecting a true null hypothesis.

Summary

What ultimately determines power is effect size, and that falls into the sometimes confusing and nebulous world of population parameters. "How big can we anticipate the effect to be" can be tricky to address. A smaller effect size requires a larger sample size, and the reverse is the case as well. What we ultimately find in our samples, which we hope represents the population at large, depends entirely on the amount of information the samples contain.

The final calculation must be tailored specifically to the statistical procedure and research methodology that is planned. Many of these calculations involve complex computations requiring dedicated software programs. This chapter merely attempts to extend your conceptual understanding of statistical power, its importance, and factors that influence it.

Nota Bene: What's Up With This "80%" Business?

The work of Cohen[1] is highly regarded in the statistical realm. His views have dominated much of statistical thinking. His classic quote, "the primary product of research inquiry is one or more measures of effect size, not *P* values," upended the traditional worship of "statistical significance" and drove the movement to reporting metrics that spoke to the matter of a measure of magnitude of any observed group differences. Cohen held to the notion that a study should have an 80% probability of detecting an existent effect. He reasoned (I will avoid the probability calculation for you) that a type I error was 4 times more onerous than a type II error. Because traditional α (*P*) significance levels are set at .05, Cohen believed that β levels should be set at .2 and power (which is $1 - \beta$) should therefore be .80. You may not embrace Cohen's 4-to-1 weighting of β and α risk, but I would not want to go toe-to-toe with Cohen in an argument on this point.

Reference

1. Cohen J. Things I have learned (so far). *Am Psychol.* 1990;45:1304-1312.

CHAPTER FOURTEEN

Can Negativity Be a Good Thing?
Implications of Publication Bias

You may have heard the tale before, one that captures the benefits of failure. Struggling through nearly a thousand experimental failures, Thomas Edison's assistants were frustrated, with one urging Edison to move on to another quest. In an interview Edison granted in 1921, he reported, "I cheerily assured him that we had learned something. For we had learned for a certainty that the thing couldn't be done that way, and that we would have to try some other way."[1]

The *Journal of Negative Results in Biomedicine* is a peer-reviewed publication dedicated to the "discussion of unexpected, controversial, provocative and/or negative results in the context of current tenets" in biomedicine.[2] Likewise, another journal, the *Journal of Negative Results*, provides a vehicle for the publication of solid science in the domains of ecology and evolutionary biology that might otherwise remain unknown.[3] Although these publications may appear as somewhat oddly unique in intent, what has increasingly been observed across a broad range of journals, including anesthesia domain–focused journals such as the *AANA Journal* and *Anesthesia & Analgesia*, is an appreciation of the importance of disseminating negative results. The bottom line is that the scientific community, biomedical and nursing journals inclusive, must avoid the bias of favoring positive trial results in the dissemination of clinical and research findings.

Consider this formalized statement of policy by the World Association of Medical Editors[4]: "Studies with negative results despite adequate power, or those challenging previously published work, should receive equal consideration." I would argue that in order for science to properly and efficiently advance, complete reporting is essential. This refers not only to the meticulous description of what was done and what was found, but also that the directionality of a study's statistical outcome does not bias its publishability. I define *publication bias* as occurring when publication of a study's findings is based on the direction or significance of the results. Although research identifying such prejudice has been around since the 1960s,[5] the actual term *publication bias* appears to have originated in a report in the social science literature by either Rosenthal[6] in 1970 or Smith[7] in 1980. Interestingly, *JAMA* once had a journal section, "Negative Results," as a monthly installment. Further investigation revealed that it first appeared in 1962 and abruptly disappeared in 1968.

The fundamental problem is that if studies with striking findings or those that reject the null hypothesis (ie, those that reveal a positive interventional effect) receive preferential treatment, substantial bias can occur should research findings to the contrary exist that go unpublished. Ultimately, this could lead to embracement of interventions that may not be justified, especially when the bias extends to meta-analyses and other systematic reviews.

Large clinical trials are extremely expensive enterprises. Quite often financial support for such studies comes from drug companies hoping to advance their product, the findings of which are custodial to the company. The "evidence" that gets advanced may be actively selected by the very industry that stands to gain (or lose) from the published results. Many recent examples of this come to mind (eg, rofecoxib [Vioxx]) that have led to the virtual universal endorsement by journal editors mandating authors' full disclosure of funding sources, conflicts of interest, and other conditions where bias may exist. Providing journal reviewers, journal editors, and journal readers with this information assists in diminishing risk associated with research sponsored by companies or organizations that have a financial or even ideological stake in seeing positive findings published.

There is compelling evidence that drug trials that show no effect or even adverse events are less likely to be published than those with positive or compelling findings. Drug companies sponsoring research must make financial gain or they will fail.[8] Highly filtered (selective) reporting, even outright data manipulation of drug trials occurs.[9,10] Bias in the dissemination of information can not only lead to promotion of unsafe or disadvantageous interventions but also may result in unnecessary economic burden.

The Funnel Plot: Gauging the Presence of Publication Bias

One available method for determining if publication bias exists is to construct a funnel plot (**Figure 14.1**). This is a graphic rendering of randomized trials that are included in a systematic review or meta-analysis. The shape of the plot can provide clues to what might be missing, such as studies that were never published as a result of publication bias. **Figure 14.2** illustrates funnel plots illustrating real-world phenomena.[11,12]

The funnel plot is subject to certain limitations and should not be viewed as an absolute indicator. For example, the funnel plot is inefficient at detecting bias when a large number of the trials that are included in the systematic review all have small sample sizes.

Judge for Yourself: A Recent "Negative" Trial and Its Downstream Consequences

The November 9, 2011, issue of *JAMA* published reports of a trial of enormous importance to those who are at high risk of stroke.[13] In this randomized trial involving 49 clinical centers and 18 positron emission tomography centers in the United States and Canada, the efficacy of surgical intervention (arterial bypass) compared with traditional medical therapy and risk factor intervention alone was assessed.[13]

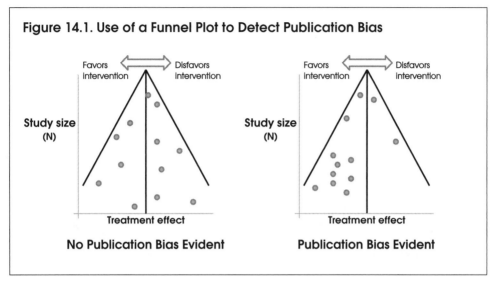

Figure 14.1. Use of a Funnel Plot to Detect Publication Bias

Although x- and y-axes can be variably represented, in this example of 12 randomized controlled trials, the treatment effect is noted on the x-axis and the sample size of the individual trials on the y-axis. Generally, the ability to estimate the treatment effect from a trial increases as the sample size increases. Smaller studies can show a wide variation in treatment effect (at bottom of plot). When there is no publication bias, the representation looks like a relatively symmetrical upside-down funnel. When bias is present, it is often seen that the smaller studies are missing, which do not favor the intervention leading to asymmetry.

This federally funded, $20 million study was brought to an early conclusion when an interim analysis revealed that the surgical intervention was not helping patients with arteriographically confirmed atherosclerotic internal carotid artery occlusion. Interestingly, this study came in the wake of another 2011 study revealing that another hopeful intervention, involving the placement of stents in the cerebral vasculature, did not prevent strokes but was actually *causing* strokes in a significant number of patients.[14]

If you have ever dealt with a faulty intravenous line, a poor arm vein, or even the plumbing in your home, you know that it just makes sense to stent, bypass, or replace the faulty architecture. In the cerebrovascular surgery realm, this logic, for all the seemingly right reasons, prevailed. In fact, when tests often revealed improved blood flow or a radiologically demonstrated larger vessel, it seemed to validate the surgical intervention. Yet the studies found that those who underwent the surgery and also received a strict regimen of drug therapy had no better outcomes than those who received the pharmacologic management alone.

Surgical intervention, especially of this nature, comes with added expense (> $40,000 per procedure) and its own constellation of potentially adverse consequences (infection, hemorrhage, tissue trauma, etc). When the surgical intervention's "costs" are compared with the long-term outcomes (quality of life, nature of long-term care, etc) of a patient who does not have the surgery and goes on to have a stroke, the surgery looks very cost-effective. In the final analysis the medication intervention alone did as well as the

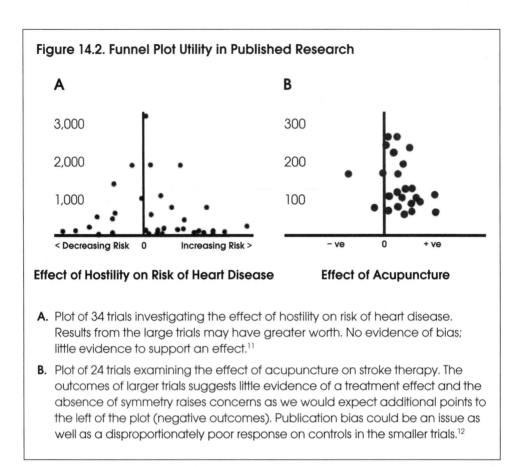

Figure 14.2. Funnel Plot Utility in Published Research

A

Effect of Hostility on Risk of Heart Disease

B

Effect of Acupuncture

A. Plot of 34 trials investigating the effect of hostility on risk of heart disease. Results from the large trials may have greater worth. No evidence of bias; little evidence to support an effect.[11]

B. Plot of 24 trials examining the effect of acupuncture on stroke therapy. The outcomes of larger trials suggests little evidence of a treatment effect and the absence of symmetry raises concerns as we would expect additional points to the left of the plot (negative outcomes). Publication bias could be an issue as well as a disproportionately poor response on controls in the smaller trials.[12]

Abbreviations: -ve, negative; +ve, positive. See Figure 14.1 for explanation of X axis and Y axis.

surgical intervention but did not, as the surgery did, cause strokes. In this bypass study, 14.4% of the patients in the surgical group experienced a stroke within 30 days, whereas only 2% in the nonsurgical group experienced a stroke within the same timeframe.[13]

The importance of the study is clear. It would be premature to assume that this intervention should be broadly applied to at-risk patients. It does not imply that it should never be used, because there is a subset of patients, as yet identified, who might uniquely benefit. It does put us all on notice that too often we may employ interventions on premature evidence and that trials that report negative findings serve to illuminate the clinical terrain in much the same ways as the results of "positive" trials do.

Summary

Publication bias, along with the common failure to report research results in ways that avoid it, creates the likelihood that biased study results abound in our literature. Although many of the causes of publication bias seem well appreciated, the enormity of its downstream consequence is largely ignored, in effect providing clinicians with misleading results at best, and at worst, resulting in widespread misperceptions and misguided interventions. The problem is not in the logistics of data analysis; thus, solutions will not be found by demanding more intense statistical analysis. Rather, the issue is the need for comprehensive reporting of results from even "negative" trials and the clear-language implications and translation of those results.

As readers of the literature seeking evidence to empower our decision making, we must appreciate that research can fail to meet its end points. Failure in research serves an invaluable role in that it steers us away from what does not work, away from lines of reasoning that may be misleading or even treacherous. As in Edison's sage take on it all, failure in research is not the problem—rather, it is the failure to recognize the implications of the failure that is important. If publication bias denies us the opportunity to gauge, and to apply negative findings should they be present, then it is the noncommunication of such failures that is the problem.

References

1. Forbes BC. *American Magazine.* 1921 [date unknown]. Cited by: Quote Investigator. I have gotten a lot of results! I know several thousand things that won't work. July 31, 2012. http://quoteinvestigator.com/2012/07/31/edison-lot-results. Accessed September 25, 2012.

2. About this journal. *Journal of Negative Results in BioMedicine* website. http://www.jnrbm.com/about. Accessed September 23, 2012.

3. *Journal of Negative Results* website. Accessed September 23, 2012.

4. World Association of Medical Editors Publication Ethics Committee. Publication ethics policies for medical journals. http://www.wame.org/resources/publication-ethics-policies-for-medical-journals/. Accessed November 15, 2011.

5. Sterling TD. Publication decisions and their possible effects on inferences drawn from tests of significance—and vice versa. *J Am Stat Assoc.* 1959;54(285):30-34.

6. Rosenthal R. The file drawer problem and tolerance for null results. *Psychological Bull.*1979;86(3):638-641.

7. Smith ML. Publication bias and meta-analysis. *Eval Educ.* 1980;4:22-24.

8. Angell M. The pharmaceutical industry—to whom is it accountable? *N Engl J Med.* 2000;342(25):1902-1904.

9. Hailey D. Scientific harassment by pharmaceutical companies: time to stop. *CMAJ.* 2000;162(2):212-213.

10. Weatherall D. Academia and industry: increasingly uneasy bedfellows [commentary]. *Lancet.* 2000;355(9215):1574.

11. Petticrew M, Gilbody S, Sheldon T. Relation between hostility and coronary heart disease: evidence does not support link. *BMJ.* 1999;319(7214):917-918.

12. Wong AM, Su T, Tang FT, Cheng PT, Liaw MY. Clinical trial of electrical acupuncture on hemiplegic stroke patients. *Am J Phys Med Rehabil.* 1999;78(2):117-122.

13. Powers WJ, Clarke WR, Grubb RL Jr, et al, COSS investigators. Extracranial-intracranial bypass surgery for stroke prevention in hemodynamic cerebral ischemia: the Carotid Occlusion Surgery Study randomized trial. *JAMA.* 2011;306(18):1983-1992.

14. Chimowitz MI, Lynn MJ, Derdeyn CP, et al, SAMMPRIS Trial investigators. Stenting versus aggressive medical therapy for intracranial artery stenosis [published correction appears in *N Engl J Med.* 2012;367(1):93]. *N Engl J Med.* 2011;365(11):993-1003.

CHAPTER FIFTEEN

Beware the Misguided (or Worse!) Evidence: Biomedical Betrayal

Some years ago, reading *Betrayers of the Truth: Fraud and Deceit in the Halls of Science,* a book by the then editors of the prestigious journal *Science,* I was astounded by their depiction of scientific misconduct.[1] Such misconduct took on a variety of forms: plagiarism, stealing others' unpublished manuscripts, and generating data from subjects who did not exist. In one extreme case, with the hope for a Nobel prize large in his mind, a respected scientist painted black patches of hair on a white mouse in a misguided effort to demonstrate the transfer and acceptance of a skin transplant without immunologic rejection. My astonishment gave way to concern as other instances of misconduct throughout the biomedical community surfaced, ultimately leading to federal and local investigations and the establishment of stringent National Institutes of Health guidelines and practices.

Misconduct Defined

I define *scientific misconduct* as the performance of a research activity in a manner that violates the validity or reliability of the findings, or engaging in conduct that violates the rights of the subjects and the integrity of the institution involved in the study. Operationalizing misconduct in this way encompasses a wide range of behaviors, from negligence to outright fraud. *Negligence* might be a consequence of cutting corners in the performance of a study or it may be a matter of investigator incompetence. *Fraud* is more malicious, involving the deliberate misrepresentation, falsification, or manufacturing of data.

Misconduct's Far-reaching Consequences

Recently attention has focused on what some describe as the most extensive pattern of misconduct in recent biomedical history, with the discovery of massive fraud by 2 well-known investigators in the anesthesia domain. In one case a Massachusetts anesthesiologist, Scott S. Reuben, was heavily fined and imprisoned for his fabrication of data involving multimodal analgesic regimens. After a letter from *Anesthesia & Analgesia* Editor Steven L. Shaefer, MD, in February 2009 announcing the retraction of 21 journal articles by Dr. Reuben, things only grew worse. A short time later an established German

146 CHAPTER FIFTEEN

Beware the Misguided (or Worse!) Evidence: Biomedical Betrayal

anesthesiologist, Joachim Boldt, was proved to have engaged in many forms of misconduct, including data fabrication, misrepresentation, and major ethical violations in his "research" on fluid therapy, with special attention to solutions of hydroxyethyl starch.

Unfortunately, these discouraging events have resulted in the application of therapies to many patients (likely hundreds of thousands) by those of us (myself included) who believed that this research marshaled important and valid clinical information to our patients. How could this have occurred? Shouldn't peer review have detected and thus prevented this from ever reaching publication? What about the saga of widespread concerns raised by research demonstrating a strong link between certain vaccinations and autism, research now known to be fraudulent yet responsible for management decisions that occurred, and likely continue to occur, worldwide?[2] And what of the remarkable case of Dr. Robert Slutsky of the University of California, San Diego, who had published 137 articles with 93 different coauthors when a whistle-blower observed some major concerns? An unbiased committee found that 77 of those papers were "valid," 48 were "questionable," and 12 were "fraudulent." In the final analysis, 17 articles were retracted, but a fog of uncertainty encompassed many of the papers in print, including those considered valid.[3] Why wasn't this appreciated sooner?

Research misconduct in the healthcare environment can cause us to stray from our search for valid (truthful) evidence, and it infects the literature like a drug-resistant organism, making its elimination extremely difficult. Once an author's work is found to be fraudulent, the profession, journal, or institution has a twofold obligation: warn us to ignore the author's findings and minimize further "infection" by other researchers and authors who may cite the paper in their work. These are not easy tasks to accomplish but are essential to the integrity of the profession's knowledge base. **Table 15.1** lists the most common reasons for a journal to formally retract a published article.

Table 15.1. Commonest Reasons for Article Retractions by a Journal

Reasons for retraction

Fraud
    Fabrication
    Falsification
    Plagiarism
Error
    Scientific mistake
    Duplicate publication
    Ethical violations
    Unstated reasons
    Journal error

Retraction of an article by a journal is the most serious sanction that can be applied to an author's work. Fabrication is the manufacture of data that does not exist in reality. Falsification is the deliberate alteration or misrepresentation of real data.

CHAPTER FIFTEEN 147

Beware the Misguided (or Worse!) Evidence: Biomedical Betrayal

Limitations of Oversight and Peer Review

We are fortunate in that the United States is one of just a handful of countries worldwide that has a bureaucratic system for evaluating alleged misconduct. The Office of Scientific Integrity was established by the US Congress in 1989 and later renamed the Office of Research Integrity. Of note is that although this office oversees work supported by the US Department of Health and Human Services, its influence is felt elsewhere. My own university, as an example, must investigate all allegations of research misconduct in federally supported research in order to meet the criteria for receiving funding. This standard is now a general one, and the same administrative process extends to all research misconduct regardless of funding source.

Readers are likely very familiar with the process and intent of peer review in scholarly and clinical publication. It serves as a kind of gatekeeper mechanism such that only research work that is performed ethically and soundly and advances our understanding in a valid and reliable manner is made formally available to the professional community. Although not a perfect process, it is generally well regarded. Your clinical and scholarly journal, the *AANA Journal,* is an example of one that employs peer review, a process that has been in existence for at least 2 centuries of biomedical journal publishing. Peer review ideally provides an unbiased appraisal of submitted work, providing critical feedback to the authors. Although clearly judgmental in nature, the process is intended to be constructive. Under most circumstances, the reviewers and editors do not have access to the actual data used, nor were they present to observe the experiment or the writing. Basic science and clinical researchers have a moral and ethical imperative to be honest and open in their work and in the dissemination of their findings. Unfortunately, the peer review process may not detect sociopathic, misguided, and otherwise unscrupulous researchers and authors. Only when other investigators find egregiously different findings in subsequent research, or when new information emerges (such as from a whistle-blower or when an institutional panel notes a concern), is research fraud detected.

My experience as Editor-in-Chief of the *AANA Journal* for more than 2 decades has only rarely brought me face-to-face with misconduct. When I have encountered it, it has usually taken on 1 of 3 broad types: plagiarism, improper authorship (ghost writing, an author listed who does not meet the threshold to be listed as such), and failure to achieve (or adequately inform) institutional review board approval. I can definitively say that editors of biomedical journals do not have the legal expertise, time, resources, or finances to secure evidence and spend the necessary months (or years) to deal with the process of managing misconduct. Consider that such a process involves collecting evidence, interviewing relevant parties, adjudicating appeals, and censoring offenders. What we can do is publish a retraction notice, inform PubMed, Cumulative Index to Nursing & Allied Health Literature (CINAHL), and other indexing sites of the matter, and learn from the experience. It is essential that journal editors play whatever active, focused role they can in repairing the damage done by an author's fraudulent work.

Research fraud generally goes undetected for a long time (often years) because the perpetrators' findings and conclusions usually make good sense. As an example we may

148   **CHAPTER FIFTEEN**

Beware the Misguided (or Worse!) Evidence: Biomedical Betrayal

believe, even observe that a drug has a certain beneficial effect when we use it a certain way. This is the very phenomenon that delayed our recognition that both Reuben and Boldt committed fraud, given that their "research findings" seemed to validate what we already seemed to know. As heinous as this is, it is made all the worse knowing that patients were placed at risk of being exposed to interventions that may be inferior (or ineffective) at best or in the worse case, exposed to interventions that may be harmful to them. With respect to Reuben and Boldt, we believe that many patients were harmed in that they were exposed to therapies that were inadequate (at best) and discouraged the use of interventions known to be effective.

The Etiology of Misconduct

It seems reasonable to ask why some researchers engage in misconduct. Is it self-aggrandizement, competition with peers, greed, ego, need for notoriety, or simply a deviant frame of mind that defies rational explanation? I once attended a *mea culpa* lecture by someone who lost her job for committing fraud, and she suggested that it was like an athlete who cheats with performance-enhancing drugs. She described such behavior as "the scientist on roids" (**Figure 15.1**). Although I was unmoved by her explanation, it is hard to know, without climbing into the heads of the perpetrators, what precisely motivates such an individual. Clearly, this is an area ripe for formal study, as little (other than editorial speculation) formalized study of the psychology of these individuals has been accomplished.

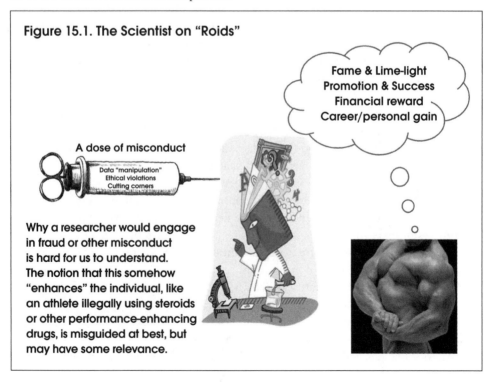

Figure 15.1. The Scientist on "Roids"

Fame & Lime-light
Promotion & Success
Financial reward
Career/personal gain

A dose of misconduct

Data "manipulation"
Ethical violations
Cutting corners

Why a researcher would engage in fraud or other misconduct is hard for us to understand. The notion that this somehow "enhances" the individual, like an athlete illegally using steroids or other performance-enhancing drugs, is misguided at best, but may have some relevance.

CHAPTER FIFTEEN   149

Beware the Misguided (or Worse!) Evidence: Biomedical Betrayal

Misconduct in Biomedical Research: Increasing or Decreasing?

I would like to end this chapter on a positive note but instead must confront the "evidence" that fraud and misconduct may actually be on the rise (**Figure 15.2**). Or perhaps we are just more aware of the possibility and our ability to detect misconduct has improved. In 2001 the number of retractions listed in PubMed for reasons of scientific fraud was in the single digits; in 2009 the number was greater than 50.[4] Also, the active physician and venerable editor of the *New England Journal of Medicine* soberingly wrote:

> It is simply no longer possible to believe much of the clinical research that is published, or to rely on the judgment of trusted physicians or authoritative medical guidelines. I take no pleasure in this conclusion, which I reached slowly and reluctantly over my two decades as editor of the *New England Journal of Medicine.*[5]

Returning to the Reuben saga mentioned at the start of this chapter, his volume of papers was so extensive over a 12-year period—we still are not completely sure what percentage of his "patient population" was real—that many of his patients were likely undermedicated for their perioperative pain. Because his work was widely referenced and imported into many review articles, his deceit likely has resulted in large numbers of patients at many different hospitals worldwide receiving analgesic regimens that were inadequate. In fact, in a study similar to one of Reuben's, a very concerning high rate of chronic postoperative pain was experienced using Reuben's multimodal recipe.[6] Because Reuben's work is so highly cited (as is Boldt's) and thus embedded in our clinical and research literature, I have grave concerns that there may be others who may see this as a recipe for their own deviant purposes.

Figure 15.2. Number of Retracted Articles (for Misconduct) Cited in PubMed, 2000-2009

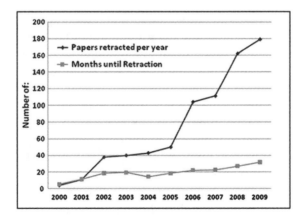

The darker line shows the number of papers listed as retracted by PubMed by year. The average time (in months) until the retraction occurred is shown by the lighter line.

150   CHAPTER FIFTEEN

Beware the Misguided (or Worse!) Evidence: Biomedical Betrayal

Perhaps my biggest concerns are grounded in the following: (1) research fraud, even when it is detected and dealt with, is usually associated with a time lag of many months to years and (2) although *hopefully* rare, we really have no idea how much fraud is occurring, as its detection is inconsistent at best. The skill of an unscrupulous researcher in defying detection must not be underestimated.

Two More Examples of Misconduct

To reaffirm and further validate the scope of the problem, I would like to offer 2 more examples of fraud and deceit in the clinical research domain. A Japanese anesthesiologist who is widely published, Dr. Yoshitaka Fujii, has produced an extensive body of work involving trials of drugs aimed at preventing and treating postoperative nausea and vomiting. Although widely published, his work has been primarily submitted (and accepted) by noteworthy anesthesia journals, especially the *Canadian Journal of Anaesthesia,* which has published at least 39 of his papers.

Careful scrutiny of Dr. Fujii's work has found widespread deception, including outright plagiarism and data manipulation and possibly data manufacturing. *Anesthesia & Analgesia,* one of the world's leading journals in the anesthesia domain, has published 24 of Dr. Fujii's papers and Dr. Steven Shafer, editor-in-chief of the prestigious journal, noted that subsequent analysis (after publication scrutiny) resulted in the view that there is "a very high probability of fraudulent data."[7]

Journals from a variety of specialties, including otolaryngology, surgery, and anesthesiology, have retracted Dr. Fujii's work. This saga, like others noted earlier, serves as reminder to all of us, that research fraud does occur, and its recognition may not become evident until long after the reports have emerged.

In January 2012, the *Saudi Journal of Anaesthesia* noted that it had published a fraudulent manuscript. The article described a study assessing the effects of dexmedetomidine and propofol in pediatric anesthesia. As it turns out, the paper was identical to a 2006 manuscript published in *Anesthesia & Analgesia.* This is horrific on 2 counts: (1) the publication was a matter of egregious plagiarism and (2) the authors claimed to have reported a study that, in fact, they did not perform, an example of manifest fraud. This can only be described as a deceit perpetrated on the anesthesia community. The matter's severity is only amplified by the discussion of previous, widespread fraudulent scientific misconduct that has occurred at the disgraced authors' institution, the MP Shah Medical College in Jamnagar, India. The entire saga is well described by Eldawlatly and Shafer[8] in the June 2012 issue of *Anesthesia & Analgesia.*

Future Considerations and a Suggested Way of Protecting Our Patients From Research Fraud

Science, as a process, is largely designed to be conservative. Research findings should be validated (replicated by others) before they are applied to patients, especially when the consequences of those applications are significant. Extraordinary claims require extraordinary evidence. Evidence-based decision making, the theme of this book,

CHAPTER FIFTEEN 151

Beware the Misguided (or Worse!) Evidence: Biomedical Betrayal

requires that each of us assumes an active role in the process. As stated earlier in the book, being an evidence-based nurse anesthetist is a demanding process. First and foremost, do no harm. Await validation of research findings before incorporating them into your clinical practice, unless the evidence is absolutely profound, and it is the safest and most effective course of action.

Although I am not affiliated in any way with the University of North Carolina, I would like to refer any interested reader to its comprehensive and clearly written guidelines and policies regarding academic misconduct. The university's graduate school website will offer the reader insightful and meaningful information regarding what constitutes misconduct, and how to deal with it. This can be accessed at: http://gradschool.unc.edu/publications/ethics.html.

References

1. Broad W, Wade N. *Betrayers of the Truth: Fraud and Deceit in the Halls of Science*. New York, NY: Simon & Schuster; 1982.

2. Eggertson L. *Lancet* retracts 12-year-old article linking autism to MMR vaccination. *CMAJ*. 2010;182(4):E199-E200.

3. Engler RL, Covell JW, Friedman PJ, Kitcher PS, Peters RM. Misrepresentation and responsibility in medical research. *N Engl J Med*. 1987;317(22):1383-1389.

4. Steen RG. Retractions in the scientific literature: is the incidence of research fraud increasing? *J Med Ethics*. 2011;37(4):249-253.

5. Angell M Drug companies & doctors: a story of corruption. *New York Review of Books*. January 15, 2009. http://www.nybooks.com/articles/archives/2009/jan/15/drug-companies-doctorsa-story-of-corruption. Accessed September 24, 2012.

6. Anderson LØ, Gaarn-Larsen L, Kristensen BB, Husted H, Otte KS, Kehlet H. Subacute pain and function after fast-track hip and knee arthroplasty. *Anaesthesia*. 2009;64(5):508-513.

7. Shafer SL. To our readers. [online response in the journal *Anesthesia & Analgesia* regarding fraudulent publication related to Dr. Fujii]. March 7, 2012. http://www.aaeditor.org/FujiiStatementOfConcern.pdf. Accessed September 24, 2012.

8. Eldawlatly A, Shafer SL. Caveat lector. *Anesth Analg*. 2012;114(6):1160-1162.

CHAPTER SIXTEEN

A Voyage in Evidence-Based Practice: What Is the Value of a Checklist in Improving Patient Care?

A few years ago, I was fortunate to be part of a national work group consisting of anesthesiologists, nurse anesthetists, industry representatives, and basic scientists whose task was to develop a preuse checklist for anesthesia equipment given the technological complexity and diversity that characterize modern apparatuses. In that process of gathering evidence and applying what was found in an efficient manner to the real world of contemporary practice, there was the opportunity to engage in the principles discussed throughout this book. In this chapter, I will illustrate the application of fundamentals of evidence-based practice in addressing important issues related to the provision of nursing and medical care by considering 2 important questions: (1) What is the value of a checklist? (2) What methods should be used to design and implement a checklist? In doing so, I will frequently draw from the lessons noted in a publication related to checklist development.[1]

The questions were selected because of the high relevance of checklist design and efficacy to the practice of nurse anesthetists. For example, according to the American Association of Nurse Anesthetists' *Scope and Standards for Nurse Anesthesia Practice*, Standard VIII, the nurse anesthetist shall:

> Adhere to appropriate safety precautions, as established within the institution, to minimize the risks of fire, explosion, electrical shock and equipment malfunction. Document on the patient's medical record that the anesthesia machine and equipment were checked.[2]

Introduction to the Problem: Questions

Checklists of all kinds are used in industrial, transportation, and healthcare (**Table 16.1**) domains as cognitive aids to facilitate safe and accurate task completion. Checklists have proved effective in various activities related to performance improvement, error prevention, and risk management.[3-7] Checklists should not be randomly assembled; instead, a systematic and comprehensive approach should be performed, especially when the stakes are high in the domain of use. Checklists may represent the standard of care in domains such as the provision of anesthesia, the transportation flight industry, and the military; therefore, their effectiveness should be evidence-based. The appropriate

Table 16.1. A Taxonomy of Checklists

Checklist type	Characteristics	Healthcare example
Criteria of merit	Order, categories, and flow are essential to achieve objectivity in conclusions	Diagnosis of brain death; clinical examination
Diagnostic	Items, tasks, and criteria are based on a flowchart model to achieve conclusions	Clinical algorithms
Iterative	Items, tasks, and criteria require repeated review to ensure validity because early check results may evolve over time	Repeated measurement of vital signs during cardiopulmonary resuscitation
Laundry list	Items, tasks, or criteria are grouped into related categories with no particular order	Medical apparatus check
Sequential	Grouping, order, and flow of listed items, tasks, and criteria are essential to achieve a valid outcome	Procedure checklist

method associated with constructing and implementing clear and effective checklists should be determined.

Given this background, an evidence-based, narrative review of the literature was conducted to determine the value of healthcare checklists and to describe the method of designing and implementing clear and effective checklists. The process and its results follow.

Evidence-Based Methods

A systematic literature search was conducted using MEDLINE for the years 1966 through 2007 using the individual terms *checklist* and *goal sheet* and the combined terms *checklist and memory* and *checklist and mnemonic*. This type of approach is termed "Boolean" with the term *or* used to allow any of the specified search terms to be present on the Web pages listed in the results and the term *and* to require that all search terms connected by "and" be present on the Web pages listed in the results. Only English-language articles were sought; the search ultimately yielded 8,303 citations. Articles were then examined for their relevance to the development or implementation of check-lists. Articles were selected based on criteria including the following: (1) description of a method for checklist development; (2) use of the checklist for process improvement or clinical support, or as a patient safety tool; and (3) description of outcomes once the checklist was used in a clinical setting. No randomized controlled trials evaluating checklist development were found.

Additional sources were searched to capture relevant information from nonmedical industries. This included Internet searches with basic search engines using the search terms *checklist, memory,* and *mnemonic.*

There is a long history of checklist use in aviation and aerospace, so the literature from the Federal Aviation Administration and the National Aeronautics and Space Administration was also searched using their organizational websites (http://www.faa.gov and http://www.nasa.gov). Relevant information sources were accessed that involved any type of documentation and literature that described the design, development, implementation, and effectiveness of checklists, and research involving checklists in any field or industry. Based on preset criteria, including the overall credibility of the source, use of peer-reviewed publications, and university-affiliated or government-published documentation, 178 sources were included for the final detailed review.

In keeping with the notion that evidence can extend beyond published material, the search was further supplemented with expert opinion by contacting content experts in areas of checklist development who were approached for interview (by phone or email) about their experiences with checklist development and use. These experts included authoritative anesthesiologists, nurse anesthetists, Federal Aviation Administration personnel, and cardiologists and intensivists who were directly associated with the development and refinement of the American Heart Association's Advance Cardiac Life Support algorithms and listed as authors or contributors on those documents. These personal communications were used to further substantiate critical points identified in the literature.

Results of the Search: Benefits of Medical Checklists

Domains such as the airline industry and the military aggressively use checklists to decrease errors of omission, reduce improper implementation of procedures and protocols, and decrease human error under stressful or otherwise demanding conditions. Healthcare providers must often analyze and manage highly complex cases under equivalently demanding and stressful conditions. Anesthesia care and emergency medicine are particularly noteworthy for their requirement of rapid decision making in a complex and stressful setting, and these disciplines make use of the types of checklists and memory aids that have proved effective in the airline industry.[8,9] Examples of published checklists currently used regularly in the medical field include those for diagnosing brain death, the anesthesia gas machine checklist, the checklist for the withdrawal of life support and end-of-life care, and the FAST HUG checklist.[7,10-13] FAST HUG is the mnemonic for *f*eeding, *a*nalgesia/sedation, *t*hrombosis prophylaxis, *h*ead of the bed elevated, *u*lcer prophylaxis, and glucose levels. This is an example of a mnemonic-driven mental checklist designed to review and prompt essential aspects of care for critically ill patients. The use of checklists and memory aids in clinical pathways has been shown to improve both the quality of care and patient safety.[4,14]

The search revealed that implementation of checklists is not always directly correlated with measurable improvements in patient care or decreases in human error; however, there was nothing found that suggested that the use of checklists actively contributed to adverse events. Examples of hazards that were considered in advance of the review included issues such as imposing an unnecessary burden on healthcare providers and delaying treatment because of using lengthy or cumbersome checklists. Instead, what emerged from the review of the literature was that a well-designed checklist compresses a large volume of essential information in a practical and convenient manner, reducing the frequency of errors of omission, and improving quality standards and the use of best practices.[15]

There are cases in which excessive use of checklists could become a hindrance. If each detail of every task was targeted for the development of a checklist, busy clinicians might experience checklist fatigue, becoming overburdened with completing these lists to the point that the lists become a hindrance to patient care. Rather than fulfilling their role as a support resource and error-management tool, checklists could unnecessarily complicate processes and decrease reliability by adding a secondary layer of complexity. To suggest strict adherence to checklists in all situations is impractical, and to do so could compromise the efficacy of a clinical process or procedure and risk infringing on efficient clinical judgment. Careful selection of checklist items and use of clinical judgment in the design of a checklist go a long way in minimizing the associated risks.

The evidence is strong that checklists are important and practical approaches to promote consistency in providing a high standard of care. The implementation of checklists for inpatients admitted because of acute myocardial infarction or stroke results in improvements in compliance with evidence-based interventions such as administration of aspirin and β-blockers early in the course of admission for myocardial infarction and administration of aspirin or clopidogrel early in the course of admission for patients having an ischemic stroke.[5]

Describing the Method for Checklist Development

A checklist is simply a list of tasks or behaviors arranged in a consistent and rational manner, allowing the user to record the presence or absence of the individual items or steps listed. Mnemonic checklists are typically used as a reminder system to help standardize normal, abnormal, or complex procedures by calling to mind items, tasks, or behaviors typically omitted during periods of stress or crisis. The benefit of using well-developed mnemonic devices is that they provide an organizational framework for quick recall of critical information and practices supported by evidence from multiple sources.[15]

Other resources with a similar goal include clinical practice guidelines, standardized order sets, and preprinted protocols or flowcharts. Clinical practice guidelines provide a benchmark of what evidence-based practice should be, and protocols systematically describe a precise and detailed plan or process. Flowcharts are a kind of diagnostic and treatment checklist in which a particular path is followed to best reach a particular outcome. Such tools typically serve the more direct purpose of memory recall and may be more appropriate for certain discrete tasks. In 2008, a colleague and I reported a study in which we performed a randomized controlled trial using an electronic checklist to facilitate evidence-based decision making in simulated, complex situations involving the anesthesia care of patients whose outcome was in jeopardy; the results revealed the efficacy of such a checklist.[16]

What Should a Checklist Look Like?

The goal of the checklist will define its structure and content. Checklists can be designed to initiate a defined action, such as checklists used in aviation and anesthesia to standardize a system's setup or in case emergency correction of an error is warranted. Such checklists are commonly used to facilitate the identification of errors of omission, helping to ensure that each checkpoint is completed appropriately, with the ultimate goal of properly setting up a system or correcting an error.

Checklists may be designed to require the participation of more than 1 person at the same time, such as checklists currently used in the domain of passenger flight. Discussion periodically arises in our literature about using dual checkout with respect to an anesthesia apparatus, but this is usually discounted because of onerous logistical issues. Dual checkout is mandated before blood transfusion to minimize the risk of administration to the incorrect patient.

Designing a Checklist Based on the Evidence

The essential ingredients necessary for designing effective checklists include basic requirements for context, content, structure, images, and usability.[17-20] Formatting-related issues include ensuring that all content in the document is evidence based, using a consistent writing style, and ensuring that the checklist is properly organized based on its ultimate goal.[21,22] Guidelines on visual effectiveness include selecting appropriate graphics, balancing the number and placement of visual elements, and appropriate use of colors, shading, and textual elements. Other important considerations outlined by key checklist developers included readability, use of familiar nomenclature, and close consideration of the expertise of eventual users throughout the development process.

Medical checklists require specific considerations for successful formatting, as listed in **Table 16.2**. It is important when formatting a medical checklist, that real-time user activities be factored into the design. Because a clinician may use a particular checklist under emergency conditions to help recall critical steps of an infrequently used procedure, the information must be straightforward and representative of routine clinical practice. This was the key theme in our anesthesia-based randomized controlled trial that used an electronic checklist.[16]

Because there is relatively little published information about the methodologic development of healthcare-specific checklists, expert opinion from members of the aeronautic, medical, and academic communities proved invaluable in helping to elucidate the approach used in designing checklists for the healthcare environment. Although the processes outlined in the literature and expert consensus can be applied to the

Table 16.2. Considerations for Formatting a Medical Checklist

Criterion	Relevant issues
Context	Where will the checklist be kept? If in a medical record, institutional regulatory body approval will be required.
Content	Evidence-based and supported by high-quality publications.
	Reflects institutional policies and procedures.
Structure	Logical and functional order consistent with real-time clinical practice.
	Consider sign-off box indicating that checklist was completed and dated.
Graphics	To improve user-friendliness; should be bold and clear.
	When appropriate, include institutional logo or letterhead consistent with other institutional documents.
Usability	Should not be overly demanding of time (ie, not onerous).
	Should not interfere with provision of patient care.
	Should use terms and phrases common to the intended domain.
	Should be piloted in advance by ultimate users.
	Should be validated, initially and at regular intervals, in its world of use.
	Should include tasks of essential importance but allow some autonomy.

development of checklists in any field, there are particular considerations when creating a checklist for use by healthcare professionals, including the following:

- Time required to use the checklist must be feasible and practical and must not interfere with the time for provision of appropriate and safe patient care.
- The checklists must be approved by appropriate administrative or regulatory authorities.
- Checklists should be reviewed frequently to reflect updates in evidence-based practice, published guidelines, and institutional policies and procedures.
- Checklists should focus on key areas or tasks commonly prone to error or omission, so as to improve accuracy, adherence to best practice, and overall process reliability.

Final Considerations Based on Best Available Evidence

Regardless of the systematic approach used to design and develop the perfect checklist, there are subsequent measures that, if not considered, could jeopardize the implementation of the checklist into practice. For example, users must be properly trained in the use of the checklist to achieve optimal results. Users must also have a full understanding of the checklist's purpose so that it is viewed as a worthy supplement to practice and not just an administrative chore. The checklist must be extensively pilot tested, ideally in simulated clinical environments and among the population of intended users, to evaluate efficacy and practicality and to assess the overall need for the checklist. Checklist designers should also consider developing an educational plan that introduces the main concepts of the checklist to the candidate users, in combination with a promotional plan to increase awareness and importance of the checklist.

Conclusion and Implementation of a Best-Evidence Approach

Checklists can serve as important tools for decreasing healthcare-related error and improving overall standards of patient care, particularly during stressful conditions when memory, vigilance, and cognitive functions can be affected. Checklists come in a variety of forms; the setting in which the checklist is to be used is a major determinant of how it should look (see Table 15.1). The development of an effective checklist involves important steps that should be systematic. Legitimacy of the content will depend on the process for its development and should include a thorough review and evaluation of the literature, evaluation of current practices, consideration of expert consensus, and a thorough validation of the checklist in the target user population before implementation of the final document (pilot testing). Checklist development should not be static; instead, it should be an ongoing process involving expert groups, up-to-date literature, and feedback from the intended users. The items contained in the final checklist represent a consensus among all members of the team and improve implementation and uptake of a checklist into daily practice.[23] The most recent global example of this in the anesthesia domain is the 2008 guidelines for the preanesthesia machine checkout procedure that was introduced because of the technological advancements and associated evolution of the anesthesia gas machine.[24]

Few studies outlined the method and special considerations for developing medical-specific checklists; this has likely contributed to their continued absence in several key fields of healthcare, despite evidence of their fundamental role in error management. Further research in the use of checklists should focus on the evaluation of checklist fatigue in healthcare, the continued evaluation of outcome improvements, and tracking of error rates. The domain of anesthesia care has generally embraced the use of checklists, but their use is still fraught with problems, in part because of the diversity of anesthesia apparatuses, inconsistent educational approaches, and resistance by some to incorporate checklists into their daily routine.[25]

Nota Bene: World Health Organization Checklist

It is estimated that more than 234 million surgical operations are performed worldwide each year, an astounding number that is believed to exceed the yearly number of childbirths.[26] Operative complications represent a formidable challenge to the global healthcare system because they represent major causes of disability and death worldwide.[27]

A 19-item surgical checklist was developed that targets the prevention of surgically related complications and is amenable to worldwide application; its efficacy was assessed in a prospective interventional study.[28] The tool incorporates dimensions of anesthesia care as well. The performance of the surgical safety checklist was studied in 8 hospitals in disparate geographic locations (Canada, India, Jordan, New Zealand, the Philippines, Tanzania, United Kingdom, and the United States). A clinically and statistically significant decline in deaths and overall surgical complications occurred after introduction of the checklist in 8 hospital sites in diverse global locations.

The World Health Organization checklist targets 3 vital timeframes during the surgical care of patients: before the start of anesthesia, before the skin incision, and before the patient departs the operating room (**Figure 16.1**). Many of the components of the checklist are already performed routinely in US hospitals, yet they had not been implemented or measured systematically. The primary focus is on team communication and ensuring that members of the team perform what is on the checklist. The items on the checklist are firmly grounded in evidence-based patient safety principles and require only a few minutes to complete.

This World Health Organization checklist is an example of a systematically derived, evidence-based tool whose intent is to improve efficacy, enhance safety, and generate better outcomes in the complex, demanding, and risky domain of global surgical care. Readers are encouraged to explore this checklist tool and consider its potential in preventing surgical complications.

Figure 16.1. WHO's Surgical Safety Checklist[28]

World Health Organization

SURGICAL SAFETY CHECKLIST (FIRST EDITION)

Before induction of anaesthesia ▸▸▸▸▸▸▸▸▸▸ Before skin incision ▸▸▸▸▸▸▸▸▸▸▸▸▸▸▸ Before patient leaves operating room

SIGN IN

- ☐ **PATIENT HAS CONFIRMED**
  - IDENTITY
  - SITE
  - PROCEDURE
  - CONSENT
- ☐ **SITE MARKED/NOT APPLICABLE**
- ☐ **ANAESTHESIA SAFETY CHECK COMPLETED**
- ☐ **PULSE OXIMETER ON PATIENT AND FUNCTIONING**

DOES PATIENT HAVE A:

KNOWN ALLERGY?
- ☐ NO
- ☐ YES

DIFFICULT AIRWAY/ASPIRATION RISK?
- ☐ NO
- ☐ YES, AND EQUIPMENT/ASSISTANCE AVAILABLE

RISK OF >500ML BLOOD LOSS (7ML/KG IN CHILDREN)?
- ☐ NO
- ☐ YES, AND ADEQUATE INTRAVENOUS ACCESS AND FLUIDS PLANNED

TIME OUT

- ☐ **CONFIRM ALL TEAM MEMBERS HAVE INTRODUCED THEMSELVES BY NAME AND ROLE**
- ☐ **SURGEON, ANAESTHESIA PROFESSIONAL AND NURSE VERBALLY CONFIRM**
  - PATIENT
  - SITE
  - PROCEDURE

ANTICIPATED CRITICAL EVENTS

- ☐ **SURGEON REVIEWS:** WHAT ARE THE CRITICAL OR UNEXPECTED STEPS, OPERATIVE DURATION, ANTICIPATED BLOOD LOSS?
- ☐ **ANAESTHESIA TEAM REVIEWS**: ARE THERE ANY PATIENT-SPECIFIC CONCERNS?
- ☐ **NURSING TEAM REVIEWS:** HAS STERILITY (INCLUDING INDICATOR RESULTS) BEEN CONFIRMED? ARE THERE EQUIPMENT ISSUES OR ANY CONCERNS?

HAS ANTIBIOTIC PROPHYLAXIS BEEN GIVEN WITHIN THE LAST 60 MINUTES?
- ☐ YES
- ☐ NOT APPLICABLE

IS ESSENTIAL IMAGING DISPLAYED?
- ☐ YES
- ☐ NOT APPLICABLE

SIGN OUT

NURSE VERBALLY CONFIRMS WITH THE TEAM:

- ☐ **THE NAME OF THE PROCEDURE RECORDED**
- ☐ **THAT INSTRUMENT, SPONGE AND NEEDLE COUNTS ARE CORRECT** (OR NOT APPLICABLE)
- ☐ **HOW THE SPECIMEN IS LABELLED** (INCLUDING PATIENT NAME)
- ☐ **WHETHER THERE ARE ANY EQUIPMENT PROBLEMS TO BE ADDRESSED**
- ☐ **SURGEON, ANAESTHESIA PROFESSIONAL AND NURSE REVIEW THE KEY CONCERNS FOR RECOVERY AND MANAGEMENT OF THIS PATIENT**

THIS CHECKLIST IS NOT INTENDED TO BE COMPREHENSIVE. ADDITIONS AND MODIFICATIONS TO FIT LOCAL PRACTICE ARE ENCOURAGED.

(Reprinted with permission from the World Health Organization (WHO), 2009.)

References

1. Hales B, Terblanche M, Fowler R, Sibbald W. Development of medical checklists for improved quality of patient care. *Int J Qual Health Care.* 2008;20(1):22-30.

2. American Association of Nurse Anesthetists. *Scope and Standards for Nurse Anesthesia Practice.* Park Ridge, IL: AANA, 2007. http://www.aana.com/uploadedFiles/Resources/Practice_Documents/scope_stds_nap07_2007.pdf. Accessed May 15, 2009.

3. Boorman DJ. Today's electronic checklists reduce likelihood of crew errors and help prevent mishaps. *Int Civil Aviat Organ J.* 2001;1:17-22.

4. Helmreich RL. On error management: lessons from aviation. *BMJ.* 2000;320(7237):781-785.

5. Wolff AM, Taylor SA, McCabe JF. Using checklists and reminders in clinical pathways to improve hospital inpatient care. *Med J Aust.* 2004;181(8):428-431.

6. Pronovost P, Needham D, Berenholtz S, et al. An intervention to decrease catheter-related bloodstream infections in the ICU. *N Engl J Med.* 2006; 355(26):2725-2732.

7. March MG, Crowley JJ. An evaluation of anesthesiologists' present checkout methods and the validity of the FDA checklist. *Anesthesiology.* 1991;75(5):724-729.

8. Liang BA. Flying lessons (special report: medical errors). *South Calif Physician.* May 2005;23-25.

9. Harrahill M, Bartkus E. Preparing the trauma patient for transfer. *J Emerg Nurs.* 1990;16(1):25-28.

10. Young GB, Frewen T, Barr HW, et al. Checklist for diagnosis of brain death [letter]. *Can J Neurol Sci.* 1991;18(1):104.

11. Runciman WB, Webb RK, Klepper ID, Lee R, Williamson JA, Barker L. The Australian Incident Monitoring Study. Crisis management—validation of an algorithm by analysis of 2000 incident reports. *Anaesth Intensive Care.* 1993;21(5):579-592.

12. Hall RI, Rocker GM, Murray D. Simple changes can improve conduct of end-of-life care in the intensive care unit. *Can J Anaesth.* 2004;51(6):631-636.

13. Vincent JL. Give your patient a FAST HUG [at least] once a day. *Crit Care Med.* 2005;33(6):1225-1229.

14. Walsh TS, Dodds S, McArdle F. Evaluation of simple criteria to predict successful weaning from mechanical ventilation in intensive care patients. *Br J Anaesth.* 2004;92(6):793-799.

15. Scriven M. *The Logic and Methodology of Checklists* [dissertation]. Claremont, CA: Claremont Graduate University; 2000.

16. Coopmans VC, Biddle C. CRNA performance using a handheld, computerized, decision-making aid during critical events in a simulated environment: a methodological inquiry. *AANA J.* 2008;76(1):29-35.

17. Bichelmeyer BA. *Checklist for Formatting Checklists.* Kalamazoo, MI: Western Michigan University Evaluation Center; 2003.

18. Stufflebeam DL. *The Checklists Development Checklist.* Kalamazoo, MI: Western Michigan University Evaluation Center; 2000.

19. Simpson SQ, Peterson DA, O'Brien-Ladner AR. Development and implementation of an ICU quality improvement checklist. *AACN Adv Crit Care.* 2007;18(2):183-189.

20. Corbin M, DeRespinis F. An approach to quality technical information: outlining nine quality characteristics. Proceedings of the STC (Society for Technical Communication) Carolina TriDoc Conference; April 8-9, 2005; Raleigh, NC.

21. Hargis G, Carey M, Hernandez AK, et al. *Developing Quality Technical Information: A Handbook for Writers and Editors.* Upper Saddle River, NJ: Prentice Hall; 2004.

22. Schriver KA. *Dynamics in Document Design: Creating Text for Readers.* New York, NY: John Wiley & Sons; 1996.

23. Lingard L, Espin S, Rubin B, et al. Getting teams to talk: development and pilot implementation of a checklist to promote interprofessional communication in the operating room. *Qual Saf Health Care.* 2005;14(5):340-346.

24. Feldman JM, Olympio MA, Martin D, Striker A. New guidelines available for pre-anesthesia checkout. *Anesth Patient Safety Found Newslett.* Spring 2008;23(1):6-7. http://apsf.org/newsletters/html/2008/spring/05_new_guidelines.htm. Accessed September 25, 2012.

25. Larson ER, Nuttall GA, Ogren BD, et al. A prospective study on anesthesia machine fault identification. *Anesth Analg.* 2007;104(1):154-156.

26. Weiser TG, Regenbogen SE, Thompson KD, et al. An estimation of the global volume of surgery: a modelling strategy based on available data. *Lancet.* 2008;372(9633):139-144.

27. Debas HT, Gosselin R, McCord C, Thind A. Surgery. In: Jamison DT, Breman JG, Measham AR, et al, eds. *Disease Control Priorities in Developing Countries.* 2nd ed. Washington, DC: International Bank for Reconstruction and Development/World Bank and Oxford University Press; 2006:1245-1260.

28. Haynes AB, Weiser TG, Berry WR, et al. A surgical safety checklist to reduce morbidity and mortality in a global population. *N Engl J Med.* 2009;360(5):491-499.

CHAPTER SEVENTEEN

The Challenge of Being
an Evidence-Based Nurse Anesthetist

Although meaningful, let alone valid, indicators are elusive, it is my view that most nurse anesthetists and our current crop of students embrace the notion of evidence-based decision making as a refreshing change from a clinical landscape that traditionally seemed dominated by anecdote. Despite the collective enthusiasm for evidence-based practice, challenges exist that must be kept in mind to ensure adequate penetration into our professional practice.

"Research-to-Practice Pipeline"

In January and April 2011 leaks in the Trans-Alaska Pipeline System resulted in downstream loss of oil causing a spike in oil prices and imposing major economic and social hardships in numerous service communities. The 800-mile-long pipeline began operating in 1977 and starts in Prudhoe Bay, Alaska, the site of an enormous US oil reserve (**Figure 17.1**). Transporting the oil resource from that reservoir in a dependable and efficient manner and delivering it to the sites of targeted use is the function of this engineering marvel. Leaks undermine this process.

Figure 17.2 depicts what I call the "Research-to-Practice Pipeline," employing the metaphor of leaky plumbing to illustrate threats to the ability of evidence translating to practice. The reader will see a large reservoir (the water cooler) filled to capacity with various types of informational (evidentiary) sources. At the top of the tank is the very best evidence, the systematic reviews, randomized controlled trials, and professional societies' evidence-based consensus guidelines, followed by less rigorous sources such as textbooks, case reports, poor research, editorials, animal research, and even the occasional clinical myths that work their way into our practice from time to time. Gaining access to the evidence can prove enormously challenging when one considers the sheer volume and dispersion of biomedical publication. Consider this: MEDLINE indexed approximately 1 million new scientific publications in the last year alone. Although thankfully not all of those are relevant to the care of the anesthetized patient, it provides some metric of the informational blitzkrieg that healthcare providers are likely to encounter in "keeping current."

Figure 17.1. Trans-Alaska Oil Pipeline

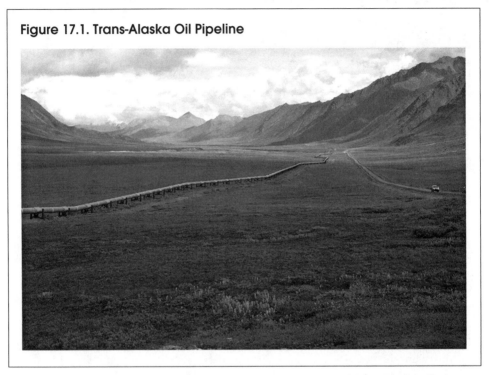

(Used with kind permission of the US Geological Survey and Dave Houseknecht, photographer.)

Phases From Evidence to Patient Care

Gaining access to the evidence is noted on the "pipeline" as becoming aware of it. This can occur through reading, attending a lecture or seminar, talking to a colleague, hearing about it through the lay media, or even having a patient mention it to us, as recently happened to me. In this latter instance, a patient I met in the preoperative holding area informed me about her sensitivity to certain opiates as well as having an unresponsiveness to clopidogrel (Plavix), and an aberrant metabolism of warfarin due to a polymorphism in her CYP2C9 isoenzyme. To my continued amazement, she described her sending a saliva sample to a genetics laboratory in Seattle, Washington, after learning of this service from a National Public Radio segment. Two weeks later her unique genetic information (relevant to pain relievers and anticoagulants) was electronically forwarded to her. Her knowledge of pharmacogenetics inspired subsequent reading and research on my part, keenly alerting me to my failure of being aware of the evidence in this domain of practice.

Even when we manage to become aware of evidence that might influence practice, we see other phases that must be transitioned through in order for patient application to actually occur. These phases (by my interpretation) include, after (1) *awareness* of the evidence, (2) our *acceptance* of the evidence, (3) our decision to *use* the evidence, (4) our *application* of it to a patient, and (5) our *adherence* to it. Along the course of this pipeline are various "leaks," which result in an erosion of evidence transference. Some of this loss is due to overt and predictable factors, whereas other loss is subject to more subtle and unpredictable influences.

For example, looking at **Figures 17.2 to 17.7**, we see that along the leaky pipeline numerous threats to evidentiary loss can occur. At each step or phase, specific factors and influences can modify the evidence that advances toward direct patient application. For example, once we become aware of information, we must consider if we accept the evidence. This, of course, depends on questions such as the following:

- Am I persuaded that the information is valid?
- Can the information be applied and thus incorporated into my practice?
- Do I have the skill set that allows me to confidently assess the information?
- How can I know that I am not considering bad or invalid information?

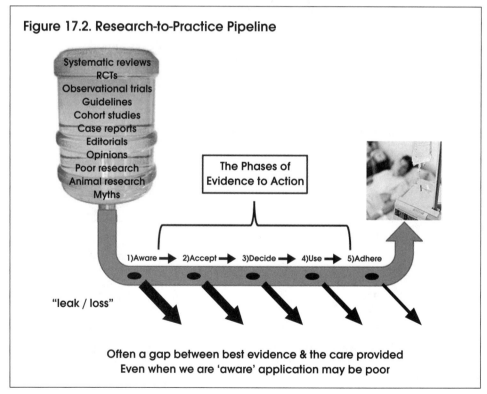

Figure 17.2. Research-to-Practice Pipeline

Systematic reviews
RCTs
Observational trials
Guidelines
Cohort studies
Case reports
Editorials
Opinions
Poor research
Animal research
Myths

The Phases of Evidence to Action

1)Aware → 2)Accept → 3)Decide → 4)Use → 5)Adhere

"leak / loss"

**Often a gap between best evidence & the care provided
Even when we are 'aware' application may be poor**

Abbreviation: RCTs , randomized clinical trials.

Figure 17.3. Why Does This Occur? Becoming Aware

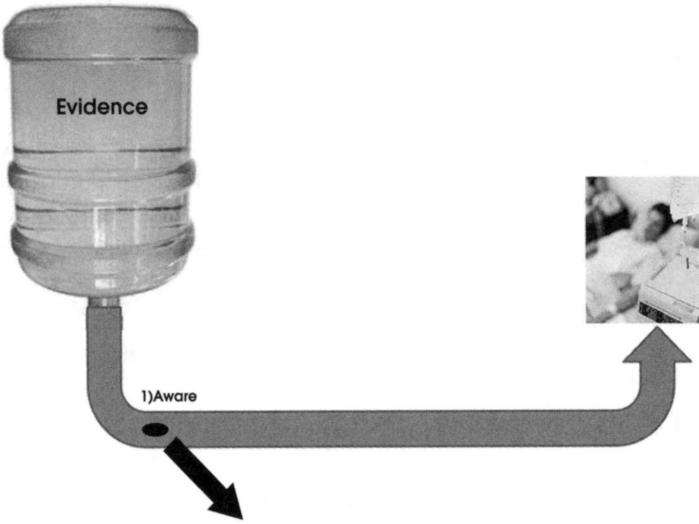

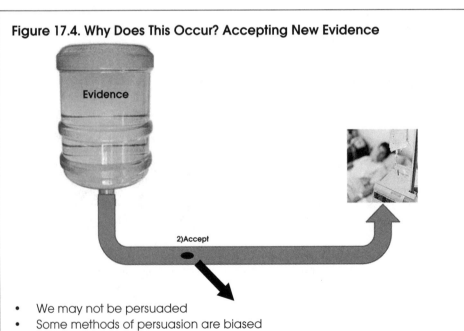

- Difficult to be aware of all the relevant and valid evidence
- Informational blitzkrieg (MEDLINE: 560,000 new articles per year)
- Exposure to evidence varies by practice locale
- Low-cost interventions may not be marketed

Figure 17.4. Why Does This Occur? Accepting New Evidence

- We may not be persuaded
- Some methods of persuasion are biased
- Some providers are not able to evaluate studies
- How can we "vaccinate" clinicians against bad evidence?

Figure 17.5. Why Does This Occur? Deciding to Use New Evidence

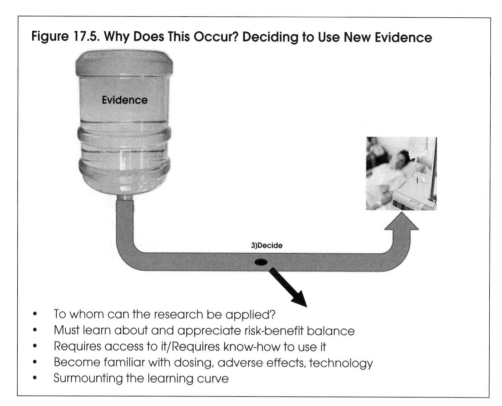

Evidence

3)Decide

- To whom can the research be applied?
- Must learn about and appreciate risk-benefit balance
- Requires access to it/Requires know-how to use it
- Become familiar with dosing, adverse effects, technology
- Surmounting the learning curve

Figure 17.6. Why Does This Occur? Using (Applying) the New Evidence

Evidence

4)Use

- Habits do not change easily
- We know, we accept, but we may forget (neglect) to do it
- Reminders (eg, checklists) may help
- May need to discuss with and educate patient: time sink[1]
- Complex mixture of attitudes, beliefs, values

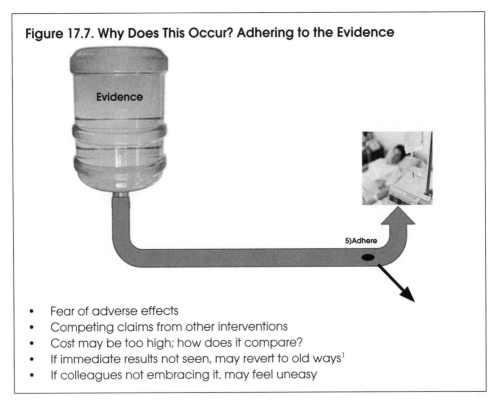

Figure 17.7. Why Does This Occur? Adhering to the Evidence

Evidence

5)Adhere

- Fear of adverse effects
- Competing claims from other interventions
- Cost may be too high; how does it compare?
- If immediate results not seen, may revert to old ways[1]
- If colleagues not embracing it, may feel uneasy

This crucial step, once navigated, is followed by the decision to actually use the evidence, creating a new set of questions that minimally includes the following:

- To whom can I apply this information?
- Am I sufficiently informed about the risks of adverse events vs the perceived benefit?
- Do I have access to this intervention (or drug)?
- Do I have the know-how to apply or use it?
- What is the learning curve associated with it, and what is the best way to surmount it?

Once I have decided to actually use the evidence in a real patient, more questions must be confronted, including these:

- Overcoming or setting aside previous patterns of behaviors or thinking
- Avoiding forgetting or neglecting to do or use the "new" evidence
- Considering the use of checklists or other reminders to help me remember
- Being thoughtful about what information (or education) I need to provide to the patient
- Dealing with patient-provider attitudes, beliefs, and values about the "new" approach

Finally comes the phase of adherence to the evidence (ie, remaining compliant with it), with questions such as this list:

- What is my concern with known and unknown (yet unidentified) adverse effects?
- How will I deal with competing "claims" of success from other interventions?
- How expensive is the application of the new evidence? Can the patient afford it?
- If superiority (over older approaches) is not seen, will I revert to the previous way?
- If my colleagues are not on board (if they don't change practice), will I continue with it?

Penetrance of Evidence Into Practice

At each of these steps, it is inevitable, for a variety of reasons, that some transference of information (evidence) will be lost, as depicted with the leaky pipe metaphor. Consider the "best case" scenario where 90% of the evidence is actually transferred across each of the 5 noted steps: from the beginning (evidence reservoir), through the steps of becoming aware (phase 1), accepting (phase 2), deciding (phase 3), using it (phase 4), and adhering to it (phase 5). In this case, the evidence actually reaching the patient is about 65% ($0.9^5 = 0.65$). Now consider if the amount of evidence transferred across each step is only 70%, here the ultimate transfer to the patient is a rather dismal 17% ($0.7^5 = 0.17$) (**Figure 17.8**). Evidence often penetrates practice unevenly, sometimes unpredictably, depending on a wide range of factors.

Figure 17.8. Penetration of Evidence into Practice

Best case: Assume 90% penetration at each step leads to 60% actually translated to patient use ($0.9^5 = 0.65$)

If 70% penetration at each step = 17% ($0.7^5 = 0.17$)

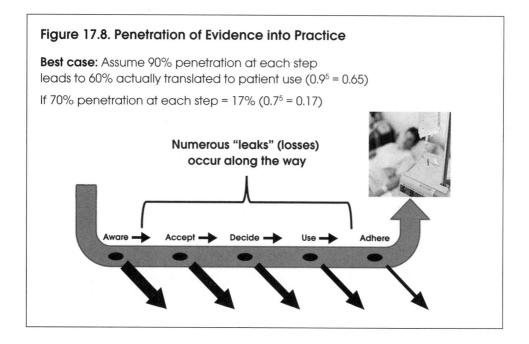

Numerous "leaks" (losses) occur along the way

Aware → Accept → Decide → Use → Adhere

Consider the enormous number of decisions that you make on a daily basis with respect to the care of your patients, and further consider what decisions are actually evidence based. Then reflect even further on what level of evidence you marshal to those individual decisions. It simply may not be practical to obtain reliable, valid and empirically sound, and cost-effective evidence for every clinical question that one has. There are always risks as well in applying any evidence to a particular patient, because in all likelihood the patient under your care was not a patient in the studies you have under consideration! The use of the PICO framework (see Chapter 2) is helpful in reducing some of the uncertainty but can never completely extinguish it.

Evidence-based practice is further complicated by what has come to be known as "indication creep."[1] This represents the practice of actively promoting the use of a drug or other intervention for an off-label indication. Examples abound. Intravenous lidocaine for suppression of the autonomic response during laryngoscopy, hyaluronidase for relief of chronic pain, caffeine for apnea of prematurity, oral transmucosal fentanyl citrate (Actiq) for treatment of noncancer-related pain, dexmedetomidine for sedation outside the intensive care unit, clonidine in neuraxial blockade solutions, diphenhydramine for sedation during monitored anesthesia care cases, and nitric oxide inhalation for treatment of sickle cell crisis are just a few examples.

Let me ask some general clinical questions where best evidence abounds in addressing them, but perhaps its penetrance is highly variable:

- What is the effect of preoperative dexamethasone on patient reports of quality of life after selected surgical procedures? What dose of dexamethasone is ideal in an adult patient and what side effects, if any, should I be concerned about?
- What is the rate of residual neuromuscular blockade in patients who received a nondepolarizer, and what is the role of quantitative tools in assessing residual blockade?
- What is the learning curve for ultrasound-guided regional anesthesia, and is it safer and more efficacious compared with traditional approaches?
- What is the rate of postoperative cognitive impairment in patients undergoing knee arthroplasty when general and regional anesthesia techniques are compared, and what are the primary factors that may influence long-term cognition?
- What happens to cerebral blood flow and cerebral tissue oxygenation when patients are placed in the steep Trendelenburg position for long robotic surgery cases?
- Does the evidence really support the removal of the antifibrinolytic aprotinin from our clinical practice?
- What are the concerns, and how valid are these, in the long-term cognitive impact of early life (neonate, infant, preadolescent) exposure to anesthetic agents?
- Are there specific genetic markers associated with postoperative nausea and vomiting and, if so, are there focused interventions that work best with individual or aggregate genetic markers?

- What is the role (if any) of potent volatile anesthetics in providing titrated, deep sedation in mechanically ventilated patients in the intensive care unit?
- What is the role of epidural anesthesia and analgesia in patients undergoing cardiac surgery? Are we too focused on proving changes in morbidity and mortality? Are outcomes studies of quality-of-life better metrics to study in these cases?
- What are the risks associated with blood transfusion therapy, and how can they best be modified?
- What are the promises and the pitfalls of anesthesia information management systems, and what can we do to maximize its potential in ensuring the best care for our patients?

We work (and learn) in an exciting, vibrant, and exponentially expanding professional domain. Opportunities for research to have an impact on practice are at an all-time high. The practical questions that I just posed merely scratch the surface of what is going on in clinical and basic science research in anesthesiology and suggest a need for carefully considering the evidence in addressing them. If you see yourself as a potential agent of change in your department or work setting, one model of cultural processing that you might consider is detailed in **Figure 17.9.**[2]

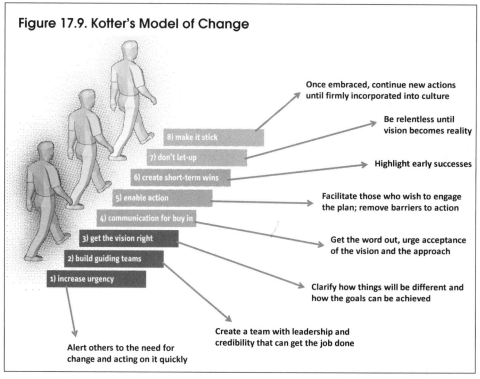

Figure 17.9. Kotter's Model of Change

8) make it stick

7) don't let-up

6) create short-term wins

5) enable action

4) communication for buy in

3) get the vision right

2) build guiding teams

1) increase urgency

Once embraced, continue new actions until firmly incorporated into culture

Be relentless until vision becomes reality

Highlight early successes

Facilitate those who wish to engage the plan; remove barriers to action

Get the word out, urge acceptance of the vision and the approach

Clarify how things will be different and how the goals can be achieved

Create a team with leadership and credibility that can get the job done

Alert others to the need for change and acting on it quickly

(Adapted from Kotter.[2])

Conclusion

In Chapter 2, I posed a question: *Do you want to be an evidence-based nurse anesthetist?* The question is admittedly somewhat rhetorical, especially if you've come this far with me! On careful consideration, a positive response to the query requires a lot from you; in fact, it is challenging to be evidence based in your care. Becoming an evidence-based nurse anesthetist means a commitment to a lifelong process of flexibility and change. Do not, as shown in **Figure 17.10**, become caught in the valley of failure to launch! Evidence-based practice is, in many ways, about a process of plugging, or at least lessening the "leaks" along the research-to-practice pipeline.

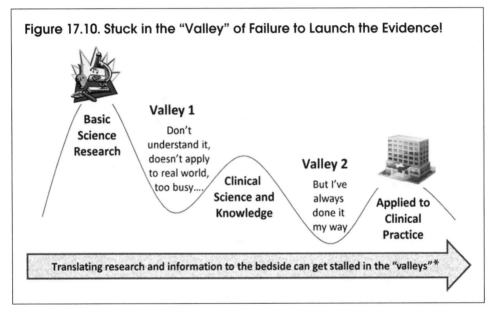

Figure 17.10. Stuck in the "Valley" of Failure to Launch the Evidence!

* Figure displays just 2 "valleys," but in some settings there may be many valleys or obstacles that stall or impede the movement of quality evidence to the patient.

References

1. Hébert PC, Stanbrook M. Indication creep: physician beware. *CMAJ.* 2007;177(7):697-699.

2. Kotter J. *Leading Change.* Boston, MA: Harvard Business School Press; 1996.

CHAPTER EIGHTEEN

Spotting Statistical Errors in Published Reports: Advanced Statistical Considerations

At the outset, it was my goal to make this a readable book for those of us (you!) interested in being an evidence-based anesthesia provider. The more I wrote, the more I realized I was merely scratching the surface in virtually all the relevant domains of evidence-based practice. Like a painter seated at the canvas, at some point in time one must simply stop and move on!

That said, I am especially cognizant of the deficiencies of my chapter on "a crash course in statistics," as the omissions are numerous and prey to criticism by those whose minds and practices are dominated by statistical processing and thinking. To that end, I'd like to add this short chapter for those who would like a quick guide to help review papers and presentations from a "statistical point of view."

Spotting Bias and Recommendations to Assist in Identifying It

As noted in Chapter 1 and Chapter 3 the primary aim of randomization is minimizing bias, although this can be an extraordinarily difficult process to implement depending on a range of circumstances. Therefore, other data collection techniques besides the randomized controlled trial will be encountered. Among these are case reports and case series, retrospective studies, and observational studies.

Observational studies are common and are generally highly susceptible to bias. One example is the so-called "treatment-by-indication" bias. Here treatments are provided to different individuals (or groups) in a study because of different clinical conditions that prevail in the individuals (or groups). Without tight control over who gets what, it may be that the subjects' unique characteristics drive the treatment and make any comparisons between or among different treatment group prone to interpretive error. "Historical controls" introduce a special kind of bias. Any new intervention is likely to show improvement, because those in the current group have probably benefited as a result of general improvements in healthcare that have occurred with time and because of the careful attention paid to them in the study.

The bias known as "ecological fallacy" manifests when an association that is observed between variables in the aggregate does not necessarily play out on the individual level. Here the details of an individual may be blurred by the group average. In general, there is great, inherent bias in any retrospective study in which there has been no control leveraged over potentially confounding variables, except for what occurs because of some after-the-fact statistical manipulation.

Selection bias is a common cause of concern as it begs to ask, "who were those guys?" This speaks to the issues related to understanding the attributes of those studied and whether they meaningfully substantiate the conclusions and recommendations for other patients that the authors generate. Keep in mind that randomized trials may select out a very special group of individuals (those who are willing to be in such a study, the special care provided a patient in a randomized trial, etc). Furthermore, the randomization process should occur with all subjects drawn from a common pool, and not as a function of gender, birth date, or their hospital number.

Equally important is for the study architects to describe how many subjects did not complete the study, and why. This is important for a variety of reasons. Was attrition due to complications? Was there an inability to tolerate the intervention? Was there investigator error in adhering to the protocol? Were there measurement failures? Were there other reasons for subject attrition that might influence our interpretation in a meaningful way? Such information is vital for us to fully evaluate the study and its implications for clinical practice.

Errors in Comparison Research

A common problem to be on the alert for is when different observers are evaluating different study groups. It is essential in such circumstances that we are informed of how the observers were prepared to perform their assessments, who they are, and a description of how well they agree in their assessments (eg, reporting an agreement coefficient such as κ). Clearly, in a study comparing approaches (eg, efficacy of 3 different procedures for achieving a successful nerve block), the observations should include each observer assessing each group. If this is not achieved, any group differences that are reported might be due to the observers and not to the intervention.

Errors in Data Analysis

In general, I become skeptical, if not downright confused, if obscure statistical procedures are used without appropriate and rational explanation. Although many may disagree with me, I believe that most clinical research studies can be accomplished with rather straightforward and common analysis procedures.

Beware, unless convincingly justified, the application of a nonparametric procedure (eg, χ^2) for the analysis of continuous data in which a parametric procedure such as a t test, analysis of variance, or linear regression would be more appropriate. The reciprocal is likewise troublesome and perhaps more common! Here a parametric procedure is being applied to data that do not reach the assumption of being normally distributed. Additionally, the dichotomizing of continuous variables (eg, blood pressure, heart rate, or serum concentration of a drug) is likewise troublesome unless the analysis is purely of a descriptive nature.

Noted previously, readers and reviewers should be alert to the overt failure to report patient or subject failure to complete a clinical trial. Clinical trials should be analyzed on an intention-to-treat basis rather than purely on a per protocol analysis, because the former will capture those who fail to complete a trial, cannot tolerate an intervention, or otherwise might be left out of the analysis.

Recognize too that tests of association may show perfect correlation, yet the actual measures may be quite different. Imagine a study designed to inform us about risks of vision loss comparing 2 methods of determining intraocular pressure during complex spine surgery. Let's assume the methods reveal an extremely similar correlation ($r = 0.94$ and $r = 0.88$) yet the actual determinations of intraocular pressure are quite different based on the method used (**Figure 18.1**). In such a study the method of Bland and Altman[1,2] would be the more appropriate procedure to employ.

Correlation Does Not Equal (Though It May Imply!) Causation

Beware the matter of the overly ambitious authors! Although all things may point to a direct, cause-and-effect relationship, only with a prospective, controlled study using specific procedures can such relationships be affirmed. Retrospective studies of any kind can only reveal strength of association, not cause and effect. Once strong relationships are discovered in observational studies, case reports, or retrospective studies, then follow-up prospective studies can be performed to seek out cause-and-effect phenomena that may be operative.

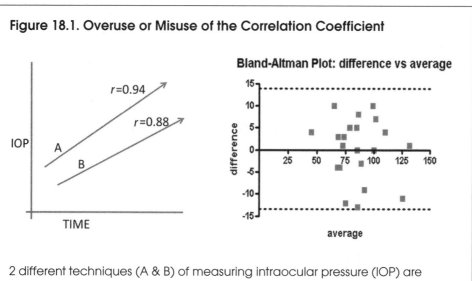

Figure 18.1. Overuse or Misuse of the Correlation Coefficient

2 different techniques (A & B) of measuring intraocular pressure (IOP) are nearly perfectly correlated yet the actual values found are quite different. This detail is lost in a simple correlation determination but nicely revealed using the technique of Bland and Altman[1,2]

Risks of Multiple Testing

Studies are generally performed—and *carefully designed*—with a specific hypothesis or research question in mind. This type of a priori establishment of methodologic inquiry and significance testing is fundamental to the systematic nature of research and analysis. Often in the analysis of data, researchers observe interesting relationships and develop post hoc subgroup or risk factor analyses. When this occurs, such relationships should be viewed as speculative or at best tenuous and in need of a more refined and primary study.

With rare exception, definitive conclusions should only be reached with formalized, a priori planned analyses of a single or at most a few absolutely clear, predefined hypotheses. Studies that go beyond this are often "data dredging" or "data mining." Although I am not implying that this is entirely pejorative, I do argue that, at best, post hoc analyses should be viewed with great caution.

There is also the risk of repeating a statistical procedure over and over. Recall that the express purpose of statistical inference is to generalize from a set of particular circumstances to a larger population from which the original cases were drawn. When one declares that "statistically significant differences are found," one is essentially declaring that the findings are not due to chance, which often is set at a less than 5% probability ($P < .05$). Problems arise when you begin to repeat the use of a test, such as a t test. Here is the concern: if one finds one or more "significant" results (using multiple tests), random coincidence can no longer be eliminated because errors may begin accruing at an unacceptably high rate.

Let's assume you have performed 20 t tests and have found that 1 reveals significance that you have established at $P < .05$. If each case, by random chance alone, has a 5% chance (ie, 1 in 20) of being significant, then one would anticipate, on average, to observe 1 significant result of these 20 tests by chance alone.

The bottom line is this: unless the statistical procedures employed are robust enough to accommodate for multiple repeats, avoid them or minimally be highly skeptical of any conclusions reached by the authors who used them.

Lastly, Does the Study Have Enough Octane?

Any study must contain a sufficient number of observations (ie, sample size) relative to the goals of the researcher. It must be large enough such that an effect, if it exists, can be determined. Although it should be large enough, it should also not be too large, where an effect of little practical or clinical importance might be statistically detected. A study that is undersized (underpowered, not enough "octane") has important economic issues in that money, time, and other resources will be wasted for lacking the capability of producing meaningful results. Likewise, an oversized study will needlessly waste resources, as more are used than necessary to achieve the goal.

Without going into the details of performing a power analysis based on effect size, study goals, and the tolerable risk of chance accounting for any differences observed, let me just say that each and every study should contain a systematic estimation and/or rationale for the sample size employed. If a rationale is not presented, the study and any associated conclusions should be viewed with a reasonable degree of uncertainty.

Conclusion: Be Skeptical—The Onus Is on the Researcher to Show Us Quality Evidence!

Assessing the appropriateness of statistical analyses can be difficult for those of us who are not extensively trained in such analyses. But a few key guideposts should be kept in mind.

- Quantitative research studies should include information in the methods section explaining how the statistical analysis was conducted and should provide a rationale for what was performed in terms that are appropriate for the journal's readership. In the case of missing data the statistical techniques that have been applied should be made very clear and any patients who are "lost" to follow-up for any reason should be clearly described in the results section of the paper.

- It is not uncommon to observe an overemphasis placed on statistically significant findings that invoke differences that are too small to be of clinical value. Alternatively, some researchers might dismiss large and potentially important differences between groups that are not statistically significant, often because sample sizes were small. Urge the use, where appropriate, of magnitude-of-effect measures that provide clinical relevance. The confidence interval (see Chapter 12) is a good example (**Figure 18.2**).

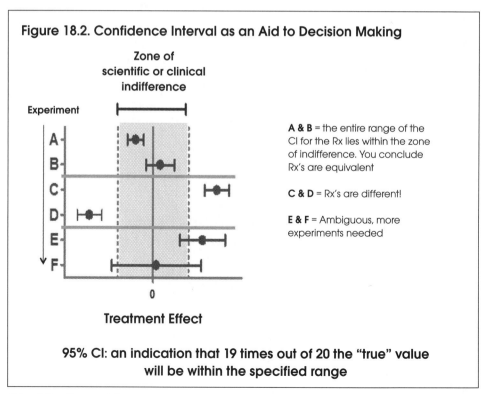

Figure 18.2. Confidence Interval as an Aid to Decision Making

A & B = the entire range of the CI for the Rx lies within the zone of indifference. You conclude Rx's are equivalent

C & D = Rx's are different!

E & F = Ambiguous, more experiments needed

95% CI: an indication that 19 times out of 20 the "true" value will be within the specified range

Abbreviation: Rx, prescription.

- Be skeptical of whether the authors generalize their findings to groups of patients or contextual scenarios that are beyond the attributes of the initial sample that was studied.
- Last, be wary of statistically significant associations that are used to imply cause and effect relationships unless those associations emerge from highly controlled, prospective cohort studies.

References

1. Bland JM, Altman DG. Comparing methods of measurement: why plotting difference against standard method is misleading. *Lancet.* 1995;346(8982): 1085-1087.

2. Bland JM, Altman DG. Measuring agreement in method comparison studies. *Stat Methods Med Res.* 1999;8(2):135-160.

CHAPTER NINETEEN

The Adaptive Clinical Trial: Implementing and Understanding the "New Kid on the Block"

Research subjects, especially patients who are involved in controlled trials, are likely to have varying degrees of discomfort in having their treatment randomly assigned. It is logical to assume that most of them would prefer to have the newer, potentially better treatment or to have their provider select what is optimal for them. Fixed assignment to a treatment in a traditional randomized clinical trial generally ignores the accumulating evidence that occurs over the course of the study, the result being that a predetermined proportion of the study population will receive what is potentially an inferior intervention. Although the primary goal of a clinical trial is to determine the best intervention, it seems logical that interim, accumulated information can be applied to improve the outcomes of study participants, especially in those subjects who enroll later in the trial.

Change While in Progress

Adaptive clinical trials (ACTs) are randomized clinical trials that allow for adaptations in the study to occur while the study is in progress. One's first reaction to this is likely fairly obvious: if one changes things during the course of the study, this violates the covenants of systematic research!

In conventional trials the safety and efficacy data are observed, recorded, and analyzed. The local monitoring agency (likely the institutional review board) examines it episodically during an interim analysis, at which time the study may be given a thumbs-up to proceed or stopped because of some compelling safety concern or when the outcome is unclear. In the ACT other options are available, namely, narrowing the study or increasing the patient population. With respect to the former, 1 or more of the initial trial treatment arms can be discontinued, and in the latter case the study can undergo expanded subject enrollment (**Figure 19.1**).

Yet another variation of the ACT is a design known as the "response-adaptive" design. Here enrolled patients are randomly assigned to a study's arms as a result of knowledge of response to the intervention in previously enrolled patients. This has been termed the "play-the-winner" design, in which patients are enrolled in those arms of the study that show the greatest promise and fewest adverse effects.

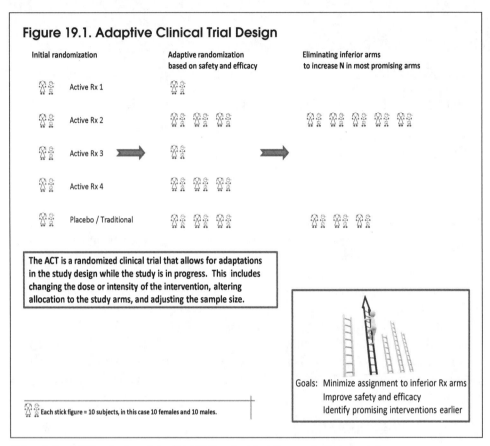

Figure 19.1. Adaptive Clinical Trial Design

Abbreviations: ACT, adaptive clinical trial; N, No. of subjects in sample; Rx, prescription.

A major benefit of the ACT design is that it allows clinical investigators an advantage in their study of the accumulating data by making real-time, ongoing adjustments to the study designed to best meet the intended objectives with greater efficiency. To maintain the integrity of the research design, such adjustments are planned in advance of the study and occur during a blinded or open interim analysis. The adjustments that can be made are many and include such things as discontinuing 1 or more of the study arms, changing or adding a study objective, adjusting allocation to study arms, and adjusting the ongoing interventions such as the dose or duration of an intervention. The ACT has great potential in drug-dosing-discovery trials, as noted in **Figure 19.2**.

Rules of the Adaptive Clinical Trial

Various rules or caveats define the ACT (**Table 19.1**). *Allocation rules* direct recruited patients to the arms of the study. Initially all recruited subjects are randomly assigned to one of the study arms. As objectively assessed data accumulates, a "play-the-winner" randomization process ensues, here subsequently recruited subjects are randomly

Figure 19.2. Adaptive Drug Dosing in Clinical Trials

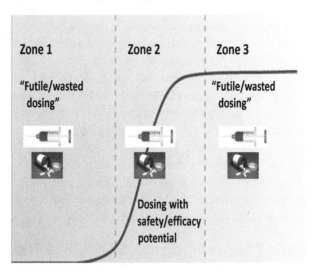

In adaptive dose-discovery trials, the dose assigned to the next patient or next group of patients is based on the response experienced by previous ones. The dose is chosen to maximize all available data about the dose response curve to measurable, predetermined outcomes. In an adaptive design the intent is to initially include only a very few patients, then focus the dosages in a range of greatest efficacy and safety.

Table 19.1. Caveats and Rules Related to the Adaptive Clinical Trial

Type of rules	Comments
Allocation	Determine how subjects are allocated to study arms
	Play-the-winner: randomize subjects successful arms
	Drop-the-loser: no assignment to poor performance arms
Sampling	Modify N (sample size) as appropriate (up or down)
	Reestimate sample size on ongoing basis
Stopping	Protect patients from harmful or futile interventions
	Enable ongoing enrollment to most successful arms
Decision	Allow for adjustments to hypothesis, outcomes, and even patient population

assigned to the successful arm or arms of the study (see Figure 19.1). The "drop-the-loser" design is just as it sounds. Analysis of early objective data can eliminate the poorly performing or unsafe study arm or arms. One downside to this approach is that studies involving dose-response-discovery relationships might be hampered.

The second caveat involves *sampling rules* that permit reestimation of the sample size (N) over the course of the study. One potential drawback here is that chance alone may modify an observed difference if this is performed too early. Careful consideration must be given to the initial power analysis performed, to avoid both type I and type II errors.

Stopping rules come into play when an arm or arms of a study are found to be inferior, futile, or associated with adverse events. This adaptive component occurs at a predetermined interim analysis.

Additionally, there are *decision rules*. Here the original study hypothesis, outcomes, or even inclusion and exclusion criteria can be altered based on an interim analysis. As an example, use of decision rules might involve modifying the patient enrollment so that any real differences between or among study arms can be better detected.

Advantages and Disadvantages of Adaptive Trials

When we encounter studies employing an adaptive component, which I believe will become increasingly common in biomedical studies, there are a number of advantages and disadvantages that clinicians evaluating such studies should consider (**Table 19.2**). Adaptive trial designs use accumulating evidence (data) to modify a particular study as it progresses without eroding the validity and integrity of the study. Although not all clinical trials are well suited for adaptive design strategies, the scientific benefits associated with traditional forms of randomization can be realized while offering trial participants a greater chance of receiving the best treatment, that is, avoiding exposure to inferior interventions. The general view is that adaptive trial designs more closely wed the sometimes divergent aims of science with the desires of patients who participate in clinical trials.

Table 19.2. Advantages and Disadvantages of Adaptive Trial Designs

Advantage	Disadvantage
Allows adjustment to increase efficiency	Challenging to maintain design integrity
Preserves internal validity	Regulatory concerns with oversight agencies
Speeds study progress	Poor understanding or unfamiliarity with design
Decreases exposure to futile intervention and adverse effects	May involve complex statistical modeling
Increases subjects' benefits to participation	May lead to misinterpretation of early data
Cost of study usually lower	Decisions may be made impatiently
Maximizes the impact of each subject's role	Overreliance on probability theory in decision making
Ideal when outcomes occur quickly in relation to subject recruitment	Necessitates resubmission of amendments to review panels (IRBs) if study is modified
Increases safety and efficacy potential	May complicate informed consent process
Identifies promising interventions earlier	

Abbreviation: IRB, independent review board.

Suggested Readings

Jahn-Eimermacher A, Ingel K. Adaptive trial design: a general methodology for censored time to event data. *Contemp Clin Trials.* 2009;30(2):171-177.

Chow S-C, Chang M. *Adaptive Design Methods in Clinical Trials.* 2nd ed. Boca Raton, FL: Chapman & Hall; 2011.

Berry DA. Adaptive clinical trials: the promise and the caution. *J Clin Oncol.* 2011;29(6):606-609.

CHAPTER TWENTY

In God We Trust—All Others, Please Bring Data: Summary, Conclusions, and Other Musings

One of the truly venerable college football coaches of all time, Woody Hayes of Ohio State University (Columbus), was once quoted as saying, "You win with people." This simplification of the process of winning has application to the field of nurse anesthesia. Clinicians and scholars do not simply and automatically appear; they must be educated and trained in the domain, and high-quality education is more important today than ever before, given the enormous, ever-growing complexity and demands of the workplace. The return (quality) on the investment (education) is proportionate in a linear and direct manner.

Coming to understand and evaluate clinical research is increasingly recognized as requiring a distinctive set of skills that are best acquired by studying and training alongside well-qualified, experienced, and passionate mentors. The current trend toward doctorally prepared nurse anesthetists will lead to more and more programs of nurse anesthesia offering high-quality didactic and practical experiences in the domain of clinical research and its application to patient care. I believe that the primary components necessary to advance the equality of anesthesia services are two-fold. First, advancing best evidence practice and second, developing strategies that refine and promote understanding on how best to marshal knowledge into practice.

Overcoming Barriers

As in other models of healthcare processes, evidence-based practice has limitations and is not yet perfect. Nurse anesthesia scholars, educators, clinicians, and students alike can, by embracing the tenets and philosophies of evidence-based practice, serve as agents of change. In particular, we need to enhance efforts in improving clinicians' access to information at the point of care, develop new strategies for communicating the evidence to patients so that they can better participate in shared decision making, and explore how evidence-based practice plays out in the real world by championing the methods of outcomes research. Are you up to the challenge?

There is still a lot to learn about what the barriers are to engaging in evidence-based practice on a routine basis. What is clear is that published guidelines and clinical trials alone cannot be relied on to change practices at the bedside. It may be that as the fundamentals of evidence-based practice are more consistently taught and actively demonstrated in programs of nurse anesthesia, its tenets will be more routinely adopted in day-to-day practice. However, more aggressive measures may be required, some that have been advocated as far back as 1981 by Eisenberg and Williams[1] and recently by others,[2-4] including the following:

- Providing feedback to healthcare professionals who adopt the principles of evidence-based practice
- Financial rewards for healthcare professionals who engage in evidence-based practice
- Financial penalties for healthcare professionals who do not engage in evidence-based practice
- Administrative changes that encourage the use of evidence-based practice
- Combining approaches, such as educational interventions with feedback
- Identifying a problem and identifying a champion of evidence-based practice to achieve its resolution

Responsibilities of Individual Nurse Anesthetists: Safety First!

Although academic centers have a hugely important role in the study of new drugs and devices, clinicians outside these centers likewise have enormous responsibility in this regard. A primary goal of industry-sponsored research is to demonstrate efficacy so that a new drug or device can be marketed for profit. As clinicians, we need to be deeply concerned about how new interventions are applied to patients at large. A new drug or procedure found to be safe and effective in phase 3 trials (**Figure 20.1**) comes with a huge price tag, helping the manufacturer recover its considerable investment in money and resources.

Nurse anesthetists often find themselves in the role of gatekeeper: the final pathway before the new intervention is actually applied to a patient. Is the intervention superior enough to existing interventions to merit the additional expense? How does the intervention's side effect profile or safety margin compare with those of the intervention now used? What does the evidence point to? As gatekeepers, if we do not ask these questions, who will?

I absolutely believe, and I stand by the overwhelming evidence in support of it, that the provision of healthcare is simply not as safe as it should be and can be. Patient safety must be engineered; it is not a passively acquired phenomenon. By using the principles of evidence-based practice, nurse anesthetists can import knowledge from the domain of human factors research, mimic behaviors and processes that define high-reliability organizations, facilitate the evolution of organizational culture, and develop high-performing teams that communicate effectively, using the latest information.

Each year the US Food and Drug Administration considers a number of devices and drugs for wide-scale distribution and marketing. **Figure 20.2** is an overview of the decision making by the Food and Drug Administration in this area for the years 2000

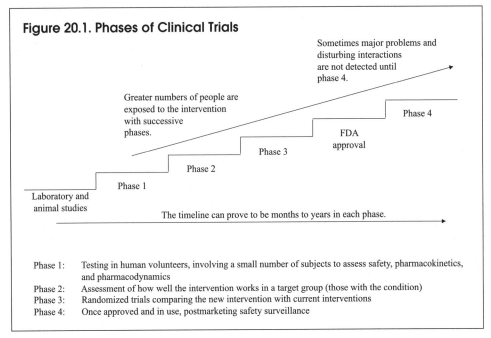

Figure 20.1. Phases of Clinical Trials

Sometimes major problems and disturbing interactions are not detected until phase 4.

Greater numbers of people are exposed to the intervention with successive phases.

Phase 4

FDA approval

Phase 3

Phase 2

Phase 1

Laboratory and animal studies

The timeline can prove to be months to years in each phase.

Phase 1:   Testing in human volunteers, involving a small number of subjects to assess safety, pharmacokinetics, and pharmacodynamics
Phase 2:   Assessment of how well the intervention works in a target group (those with the condition)
Phase 3:   Randomized trials comparing the new intervention with current interventions
Phase 4:   Once approved and in use, postmarketing safety surveillance

Abbreviation: FDA, US Food and Drug Administration.

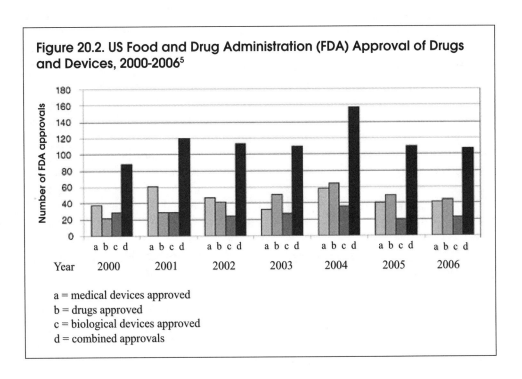

Figure 20.2. US Food and Drug Administration (FDA) Approval of Drugs and Devices, 2000-2006[5]

a = medical devices approved
b = drugs approved
c = biological devices approved
d = combined approvals

through 2006.[5] The public believes (expects) that the system will not only protect them from harm by preventing the approval and distribution of ineffective, unsafe, or unreasonably priced technologies but also will fast-track promising, beneficial technologies. There is an inherent tension, if not the occasional outright conflict, that exists between these expectations. In fact, we have known for some time that hundreds of thousands of patients (some argue millions) experience harm because of the failure to use, or to excessively use or to outright misuse, healthcare interventions of all kinds.[6-10]

Six Sigma, a term that originated with the Motorola Corporation, is a process of quality procedures and measures embraced by many business organizations worldwide; it refers to the quest to reach near perfection in its product. It represents a highly disciplined, evidence (data)-grounded method for eliminating errors and defects from the initial manufacturing of the product through the product's dissemination (marketing) and implementation (service) phases. The orientation of the "six" and the "sigma" involves reference to the statistical term for standard deviation (sigma) and to achieving the goal of being 6 SDs from the mean, which is in the order of remoteness (somewhere near 3 failures in 1 million events). Six Sigma quantitatively describes a process or a goal of an organization for minimizing mistakes using standardized, data-driven enterprises.

We are fortunate to be in a healthcare specialty that has made great strides in applying the principles and philosophies of the Six Sigma benchmark of performance. Although there is disagreement among authorities as to what is the best metric to track in quantifying risk reduction, many suggest that if mortality and persistent vegetative coma are used as surrogate measures of anesthetic safety, then the systematic, focused, and multidimensional efforts of the anesthesia community during the last 30 to 40 years have resulted in a 10-fold improvement in patient safety.

Progress in the realm of safe provision of care is due to a host of reasons, including the research and development of new drugs and techniques. Research and development of safer inhalational anesthetics, autonomic nervous system modifiers, monitoring devices, and regional anesthesia techniques represent just a few obvious examples. But overshadowing these innovations has been a concerted effort, based on importing the latest valid evidence, to advance the science associated with other dimensions of the processes associated with anesthesia care (**Table 20.1**). Concerted efforts directed at improving anesthesia safety are a priority of the major anesthesia organizations, including the American Association of Nurse Anesthetists, the American Society of Anesthesiologists, the Anesthesia Patient Safety Foundation, the International Anesthesia Research Society, and other specialty groups.

The Megacohort and Personalized Medicine: New Horizons, New Possibilities

I can marshal an argument that epidemiology has played a critical and perhaps unsurpassed role in advancing what might be called the science of the population. In the 17th century a Londoner, John Graunt, using records first established in the mid-1500s, studied records of death and identified many population trends, including male births outnumbering female births.[11] In the mid-19th century, John Snow,[12] the father of epidemiology and

---

Table 20.1. Progress in the Realm of Patient Safety: It's Not Just Drugs and Technology

Greater attention to the preoperative preparation of patients

Emphasis on tracking outcomes in the postoperative period

Advances in the organization of anesthesia services

Strict guidelines for continuing education requirements

Systematic improvements in the manner in which we educate students (didactics, simulation, program length, case numbers, faculty credentials)

Better attention to the supervision requirements of trainees

Advances in the realm of communication and teamwork science

Understanding the culture of safety in the operating room

---

also an anesthesiologist who illuminated a good deal of terrain in the anesthesia domain, saved tens of thousands of lives worldwide with his survey work revealing that cholera was spread by the ingestion of contaminated water, a conclusion based wholly on the deaths of a relative few people. Doll and Hill's[13] landmark publication in 1954 impeached cigarette smoking as a cause of lung cancer. The Framingham Heart Study established the value of analyzing risk factors using a sample of only about 5,000 subjects.[14] The first major, formally published controlled clinical trial (investigating streptomycin as a treatment of tuberculosis), occurred with the oversight of Bradford Hill, a population scientist and colleague of Doll.[15]

These landmark works set the foundation for what is going on today, and what we are all beneficiaries of. Exploring the human genome is the latest territory for the population scientist, bringing with it unparalleled opportunity (and challenge). Whether it be hypertension, cancer, infectious disease, or response to drug therapy (of profound interest to those of us who administer anesthesia), genetic analysis allows us to move beyond the assessment of risk solely due to just a few exposure factors. Instead pharmacogenetics provides investigators with an exponential leap in factors to interrogate based simply on the number of genes (approximately 40,000) that code for each us, variations in those genes, and even gene-to-environment interaction (epigenetics). The hope and promise of personalized medicine is finally upon us.

Megacohorts, resulting from the pooling of existing databases of tens of thousands of subjects, are merging with new technologies (bioinformatics) and novel statistical procedures that will facilitate the manipulation and translation of larger and larger data sets to help address, and solve, clinically relevant questions (**Figure 20.3**). North America and Europe are actively amassing a previously unimaginable array of massive "biobanks" (megacohorts). Among these, just to name a few, are the United Kingdom Biobank; the Kaiser Permanente Research Program on Genes, Environment, and Health;

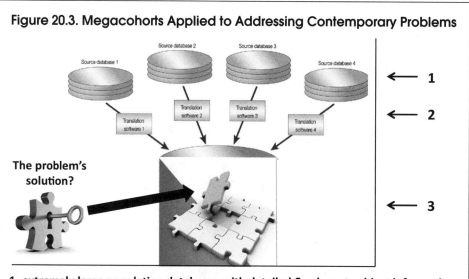

Figure 20.3. Megacohorts Applied to Addressing Contemporary Problems

1- extremely large population databases with detailed & relevant subject information
2- appropriate translational manipulation and analysis of data
3- focused attention to relevant, clinically-based problem(s) with solution(s)

and the Department of Veterans Affairs' Million Veteran Program. Each of these currently consists of 500,000 to greater than 1 million subjects, each growing by the day. The advent of electronic record keeping has made this all possible. Readers interested in exploring the possibilities of advancing evidence-based decision making (EBDM) in the domain of massive databases are urged to read the short article by Manolio and Collins.[16]

The fundamental and future direction of patient-centered outcomes research is directed at assisting us in making informed and safe decisions regarding the care that we provide. A good deal of the daily decision making that we engage in is based on observational and quasi-experimental based research. Contemporary (and future) database construction will benefit from advances in the domain of information technology that both researchers and clinicians will reap rewards from.

A recent success story is in the realm of treatment of chronic hepatitis C virus (HCV) infection, something of concern to all healthcare workers. In the modern engineering of therapy, new approaches using EBDM, involve patient-specific factors such as viral genotype and early treatment responses in considering treatment approach. Using large databases of information, predictors of drug response led to the discovery that a single-nucleotide polymorphism near the *IL28B* gene strongly predicted the response to therapy involving peginterferon-α and ribavirin.[17]

Initial and follow-up studies demonstrated predictive response rates to therapy based on favorable vs nonfavorable genotype of the person with chronic HCV, providing an essential, patient-specific therapy guide. This is just one example of the far-reaching relevance of merging large databases with EBDM information, in this case, knowledge of pharmacogenetic discoveries.

Now that we are in the genomic era, patient-centered therapeutics will be better informed by information gleaned from large databases of relevant clinical and research-derived information. The story of chronic HCV and drug intervention is just one of many current and evolving examples.

Evolution and a Look to the Future

The term *evidence-based medicine* first appeared in the published literature in 1991.[18] Since that time, the philosophies and processes associated with evidence-based medicine have hybridized and evolved to the point at which it is now an internationally embraced and practiced healthcare model. Evidence-based practice is a rubric for a multidimensional model emphasizing the formulation of focused questions, a robust search and retrieval of the best-available evidence from reliable sources, a quality analysis of the found evidence to assess its validity in the context of the original question, and a careful application of the resultant evidence in the unique setting of an individual patient.

Getting to the evidence has never been easier, a function in no small part due to the development and widespread use of the Internet. The sentinel work of the National Library of Medicine in making MEDLINE databases available via its portal, PubMed, and commercial portals such as Ovid and Google, allow access to a wealth of evidence with just a few keyboard strokes. The dissemination of systematic reviews, primary studies, practice guidelines, and databases of all kinds can be obtained from other sources such as the *ACP Journal Club,* BMJ Publishing Group's *Clinical Evidence,* UpToDate.com, and The Cochrane Library, just to mention a few. Complementing these evidentiary sources is an amazingly diverse group of online electronic textbooks. These types of offerings would have been unimaginable just a few decades ago.

As in building a strong brick wall, the final product is a function of doing a lot of little things correctly. That more and more of our interventions, our processes, our approaches, and our interactions are evidence-based has, in my view, had a tremendous role in improving the care that we provide. It is important for us all to understand that once we gather the evidence, scrutinize it carefully, and weigh its value, an important tenet of evidence-based practice must still unfold. This is the inclusion of patients' values and preferences in designing a plan of care so that they are sufficiently informed and can participate as a decision maker to the extent that is possible.

In Chapter 1, I illustrated the disconnect between the needs of people and the objectives of science that Gulliver witnessed on his travels. Many of our patients trust in the system that marshals the care that they receive. Although we should acknowledge their sense of trust, we must also recognize that the best way to fulfill that patient trust is for each of us to come to the bedside armed with the best possible evidence.

So, you want to be an evidence-based anesthetist? Then be one.

References

1. Eisenberg JM, Williams SV. Cost containment and changing physicians' practice behavior. *JAMA*. 1981;246(19):2195-2201.

2. Greco PJ, Eisenberg JM. Changing physician practices. *N Engl J Med*. 1993;329(17):1271-1274.

3. Solomon DH, Hashimoto H, Daltroy L, et al. Techniques to improve physicians' use of diagnostic tests: a new conceptual framework. *JAMA*. 1998;280(23):2020-2027.

4. Lundberg GD. Perseverance of laboratory test ordering: a syndrome affecting clinicians [editorial]. *JAMA*. 1983;249(5):639.

5. Owens J. 2006 drug approvals: finding the niche [published correction in *Nat Rev Drug Discovery*. March 2007] . *Nat Rev Drug Discovery*. 2007;6: 99-101. http://www.nature.com/nrd/journal/v6/n2/full/nrd2247.html. Accessed October 7, 2012.

6. Chassin MR, Galvin RW. The urgent need to improve healthcare quality. *JAMA*. 1998;280(11):1000-1005.

7. Institute of Medicine. *Crossing the Quality Chasm: A New Health System for the 21st Century*. Washington, DC: National Academies Press; 2001.

8. Kohn LT, Corrigan JM, Donaldson MS, eds. *To Err is Human: Building a Safer Health System*. Washington DC: National Academies Press; 2000.

9. Brennan TA, Gawande A, Thomas E, Studert D. Accidental deaths, saved lives, and improved quality. *N Engl J Med*. 2005;353(13):1405-1409.

10. Berwick DM, Calkins DR, McCannon CJ, Hackbarth AD. The 100,000 Lives Campaign: setting a goal and a deadline for improving health care quality. *JAMA*. 2006;295(3):324-327.

11. Rothman KJ. Lessons from John Graunt. *Lancet*. 1996;347(8993):37-39.

12. Snow J. *On the Mode of Communication of Cholera*, 8 volumes, London, UK: John Churchill 1849; 2nd ed. 1855.

13. Doll R, Hill AB. The mortality of doctors in relation to their smoking habits: a preliminary report. *BMJ*. 1954;1(4877):1451-1455.

14. Coll R. Cohort studies: history of the method. *Soz Praventivmed*. 2001;46:75-86.

15. Medical Research Council Investigation. Streptomycin treatment of pulmonary tuberculosis. *BMJ*. 1948;2:769-782.

16. Manolio TA, Collins R. Enhancing the feasibility of large cohort studies. *JAMA*. 2010;304(20):2290-2291.

17. Clark PJ, Thompson AJ, McHutchison JG. IL28B genomic-based treatment paradigms for patients with chronic hepatitis C virus infection: the future of personalized HCV therapies. *Am J Gastroenterol.* 2011;106(1):38-45.

18. Guyatt G. Evidence-based medicine [abstract]. *ACP J Club.* 1991;114 (suppl 2):A16.

Glossary

Adaptive clinical trial: A study method allowing for design modifications during a study, with the goal of implementing the data as early as possible for the benefit of patients and the interventional development process.

Allocation concealment: People enrolling participants in a randomized trial are unaware of the group to which the next participant will be assigned.

Alternative hypothesis: The prediction that is not tentatively held to be true; it states that a relationship will be found between 2 variables or that the means of multiple groups are not equal.

Analysis of variance (ANOVA): Used to test hypotheses about differences in the average values of an outcome between 2 groups; while the t test can be used to compare 2 means or 1 mean against a known distribution, ANOVA can be used to examine differences among the means of 2 or more different groups at once.

Appropriate sample size: An appropriate sample size is one sufficient to detect a statistical difference or effect that the researcher identifies as representing a meaningful result, given that such an effect truly exists within the data, without wastefully oversampling. Too large a sample tends to yield statistical significance even in the presence of a small effect, that is, statistical significance overrides the practical significance of the results. Such a situation leads to the risk of a type I error. On the other hand, too small a sample tends to suggest that there is no reasonable effect due to the intervention; but, even a large effect can be difficult to detect if the sample size is inadequate. This situation leads to an increased chance of a type II error.

Bias: Inclusion of subjects or methods such that the results obtained are not truly representative of the population from which it is drawn.

Bland-Altman plot: A method used to calculate the mean differences between different measures of a phenomenon (eg, invasive vs noninvasive blood pressure monitoring) to determine their degree of interchangeability.

Blinding: The process by which the researcher and/or the subject is unaware of which intervention or exposure has occurred.

Case-control study: Patients who have the outcome of interest (eg, aspiration, nausea, or awareness) become the cases, and patients who are otherwise matched (eg, by gender, age, comorbidity, and surgery type) who did not experience the outcome serve as the control subjects to help identify potential contributing factors.

Categorical variable: A characteristic that has been measured on a nominal scale.

Cochrane Collaboration: An Internet-accessed source that synthesizes and makes readily available systematic reviews of healthcare interventions and promotes research designed to make the latest and most valid healthcare-related evidence available to clinicians.

Coefficient of determination (r^2): The overall proportion (percentage) of variance in one variable that is attributed to the variation in another variable; for example, a correlation of $r = 0.8$ would have an r^2 of 64%.

Cohen *d*: An effect size measure representing the standardized difference between 2 means.

Cohort study: A study of 2 or more groups (cohorts) forward in time to assess the effect of an intervention.

Condition (group) mean: The average of the scores of all study subjects in a group.

Confidence interval (CI): The range of values that is formed to contain within its boundaries, with a predetermined level of confidence, the population value being estimated. It is usually reported as the 95% CI; assuming a number needed to treat (NNT) of 10 with a 95% CI of 5 to 15 suggests 95% confidence that the true NNT value is between 5 and 15 in the sample population.

Confounder: A variable that is associated with the exposure and the outcome of interest that is not the variable being studied.

Continuous variable: A variable that theoretically can assume an infinite number of values (something that is measurable and ongoing).

Control group: A group of subjects without the condition of interest, or unexposed to or not treated with the intervention of interest.

Convenience sample: Subjects who, for whatever set of reasons, are conveniently available to the researcher for inclusion in a study, such as patients having defined surgical procedures during the study period. Random selection is, thus, obviated, but then the included subjects are randomly assigned to the study's treatment arms.

Cost-benefit analysis: An assessment of whether the cost of an intervention is worth the benefit derived.

Critical value: A value that a statistic must surpass to have a hypothesis test result in rejection of the null hypothesis.

Crossover design: A patient or patient group receives 2 or more experimental interventions, 1 after the other, in either a specified or random order.

Cross-sectional study: The observation (measurement) of a population at a single time point or at a specified interval.

Dependent groups *t* test: A statistical technique to compare the means of 2 related samples, such as pre-post differences, or analyses comparing the means of dependent pairs such as husbands and wives, sibling pairs, or twins. Also called a paired or correlated *t* test.

Double-blind study: Neither the subject (patient) nor the observer is aware of what intervention has been applied.

Double-dummy blinding: Generally used in a drug-intervention study; participants receive the assigned "active" drug and the placebo matched to the comparison drug. Such trials involve 2 active drugs and 2 matching placebos. For example, in comparing 2 drugs, 1 in a green capsule and the other in an orange capsule, the investigator would acquire green placebo capsules and orange placebo capsules. This approach is believed to improve the double-blinding process. This is also known as the "double-placebo" design.

Double-placebo design: See Double-dummy blinding.

Effect size: An index measuring the magnitude of a specific result. Effect sizes can be standardized comparisons of means, or they can be correlation coefficients or squared correlation coefficients. Effect sizes are used to assess the degree to which the research hypothesis under study is actually observed via the sample data.

Effectiveness: A measure of how well the drug or intervention works and encompasses tolerability and ease of use as well.

Efficacy: A measure of the ability of a drug or intervention to treat the condition for which it is indicated. It is not a statement about tolerability or ease of use. Something may have efficacy yet be limited because of side effects or be limited in its use because of complexity in its application (effectiveness issues).

Evidence-based practice: The conscientious, explicit, and judicious use of the current best evidence available from systematic research in making decisions about the care of an individual patient; it requires the integration of found evidence with an individual clinician's expertise and the values and desires of the patient.

External validity: Refers to the generalizability of a study's findings. It asks the question, "To whom can the results of a particular study be applied?"

Factorial analysis of variance: A procedure for comparing the mean scores of 2 or more groups based on 2 or more (categorical) independent variables; it also tests for interactions among the independent variables.

False positive: A test result that suggests that the subject has a specific disease or condition when, in fact, the subject does not.

F distribution: A theoretical relative frequency distribution of the ratio of 2 independent sample variances.

Forest plot: A display revealing a summary of the strength of the evidence in clinical trials and frequently used to graphically portray a meta-analysis of a group of associated randomized controlled trials.

Funnel plot: A graph that portrays the existence (or not) of publication bias in a systematic review.

Homoscedasticity/heteroscedasticity: Important in linear regression applications. Homoscedasticity indicates that the variability in scores for the independent variable is the same for all values of the dependent variable. Heteroscedasticity indicates that relationship is not consistent.

Incidence: Number of new cases that develop during a specified time interval.

Independent groups *t* test: A procedure for comparing the mean scores of 2 independent groups on a given quantitative variable.

Intention-to-treat analysis: The inclusion of all patients in the final analysis of a clinical trial, regardless of whether they completed or received the intended treatment, to fully preserve the principles of randomization and to fully account for subject loss.

Interim analysis: Analysis of the data at 1 or more time points before the official close of the study with the intention of possibly terminating the study early should the early analysis prove particularly compelling or in favor of or against the intervention.

Internal validity: The rigor with which a study has been designed and performed; addresses the certainty that the conclusions found can be relied on.

Kaplan-Meier curve: A technique that performs some sort of outcome, often survival analysis over time. It involves computing the number of people who have a particular outcome (usually negative) at a particular time with a longitudinal graphing to compare groups managed differently.

Kappa statistic (κ): A measure describing the degree of agreement between 2 observers who are rating the same, categorical scale variable. A κ of 1.0 suggests perfect agreement, with values less than 1.0 representing proportionately decreasing levels of agreement.

Latency: A time period between exposure to an agent and the development of the changes associated with that exposure.

Linear regression: See Regression analysis.

Matching: Process by which each case is matched with 1 or more controls, which have been deliberately chosen to be as similar to the test subjects in all regards other than the variable being studied.

Meta-analysis: A systematic review using quantitative analytical methods to synthesize and summarize the results.

Multiple regression: A procedure for determining the relationship between a criterion variable and several predictor variables.

Narrative review: A review of a topic (specific or generalized) that does not include or follow a systematic evidence-based strategy based on predetermined criteria for inclusion of cited studies. This type of review is subject to bias and interpretive issues, and caution should be applied in relying on a narrative review when drawing conclusions about patient care.

N-of-1 trial: One patient undergoes pairs of interventional periods in which 1 period involves the use of the experimental treatment and the other involves the use of an alternative treatment (or placebo). Double blinding is maintained and outcomes are assessed.

Nonparametric statistics: Sometimes called distribution-free statistics because they do not require that the data fit a normal distribution. In general, nonparametric tests require less restrictive assumptions about the data and permit the analysis of categorical and rank data.

Null hypothesis: The prediction that is tentatively held to be true; it states that no relationship will be found between 2 variables or that the means of multiple groups are equal.

Number needed to treat (NNT): The number of patients who need to be treated with an intervention in order to prevent 1 predetermined complication, such as nausea and vomiting, hypertension, recall, hypothermia, or some other negative outcome.

Observational study: A study in which no intervention is made; these studies provide estimates and examine associations of events in their natural setting.

Odds ratio (OR): A technique of comparing whether the probability of an event occurring is the same for 2 groups. An OR of 1 suggests that the event is equally likely in both groups. An OR of more than 1 implies that the event is more likely in the first group, whereas an OR of less than 1 implies that the event is less likely in the first group.

One-tailed test: A statistical test in which the critical region for rejecting the null hypothesis falls in 1 direction of the probability distribution.

One-way analysis of variance: A procedure for comparing the mean scores of 2 or more groups based on 1 independent variable.

Parametric statistics: Inferential statistics are procedures for hypothesis testing that assume that the variables being assessed follow a normal (ie, bell-shaped) distribution.

Per protocol analysis: In contrast with the intention-to-treat analysis, this analysis includes only patients who actually complete the planned clinical trial or intervention analyzed and does not include patients who dropped out of, or were otherwise lost, from the study.

PICO: A mnemonic that refers to the process of developing a focused clinical question by stating it in terms of the following essential components: *p*atient, *i*ntervention, *c*omparison, and *o*utcome.

Pooled variance: Also called "within-groups" variability. Under the assumption of equal population variances, the pooled variance represents the best estimate of this equal but unknown population variance. It is a weighted average of the variance within each group.

Population: The group or collection of people from which a sample was drawn and/or to which one hopes to generalize based on sample results.

Power: In hypothesis testing, the power refers to the probability of making a correct decision to reject the null hypothesis. Power indicates the likelihood of detecting a difference between groups or a hypothesized relationship within the population of interest.

Prevalence: The number of cases of a condition that exists in a defined population at a specific time point.

Propensity analysis: The probability of a patient having been treated conditional on the patient's background (pretreatment) characteristics. Intuitively, the propensity score is a measure of the likelihood that a person would have been treated based on his or her background characteristic. It is sometimes used to more critically assess the bias associated with an observational study.

Publication bias: The notion that studies that report a positive effect of an intervention are more likely to be published in quality journals than reports of a negative or absent effect. The resultant risk is that the extant literature may give an overly optimistic view of an intervention's effectiveness.

P value: Obtained significance level for a statistical test. The *P* value represents the likelihood, under the assumption that the null hypothesis is true, that the data would yield the obtained results. Often referred to as the "alpha (α)," a *P* value of less than .05 is traditionally chosen as the level of significance.

r^2: See Coefficient of determination.

Randomization: A process whereby all members of a population have an equivalent chance of being chosen to participate in a study (random selection); a process by which all members of a sample have an equivalent chance of being placed in each of the treatment arms of a study (random assignment).

Randomized controlled trial (RCT): A prospective approach used to evaluate an intervention's efficacy or effectiveness requiring random assignment of subjects to the study's different intervention arms. This approach ensures that known and unknown confounding factors are evenly distributed between or among the treatment groups.

Regression analysis/linear regression: Explores relationships between a well-defined dependent variable and 1 or more independent variables termed predictor variables. Linear modeling investigates such relationships that are summarized by straight lines known as "lines of best fit."

Relative risk (RR): Also known as the risk ratio, it represents the risk of an event occurring on the basis of some type of exposure. The RR is a ratio of the probability of the event occurring in an exposed group compared with a nonexposed group. For example, if the probability of a patient experiencing a sore throat after intubation was 8% and among patients who had a laryngeal mask airway placed was 1%, the RR of sore throat associated with intubation would be 8.

Reliability: Refers to the extent to which measurements are consistent over time and setting, providing accurate representation of subjects under study; it also refers to the issue of where a study can be reproduced under similar conditions.

Response rate: The proportion of subjects who respond to either a treatment (intervention) or a questionnaire.

Risk factor: A variable associated with a specific outcome of interest.

Rule of 3: Given an unknown probability (P), if no event occurs in a trial, a quick approximation of the upper 95% confidence limit for the event occurring again is $P = 3/N$. If a trial has 1,500 subjects without an adverse event, the rate of adverse events, with 95% confidence, is no more frequent than 1 in 500.

Sample: Collection of observations selected in such a way as to offer a model of the population of interest.

Sensitivity: The proportion of patients who actually have the target disorder who have a positive test result.

Significance level: In hypothesis testing, the significance level refers to the probability of making a type I error, or rejecting the null hypothesis when it is actually true. The researcher decides on the level of significance for each test.

Single-blind study: A prospective investigation in which the subjects, who have been randomized to the treatment arms, are shielded from knowledge of what intervention they are to receive.

Six Sigma: Quantitatively describes a process or goal of an organization in minimizing mistakes using standardized, data-driven enterprises. It refers to being 6 SDs from the mean, the idea being that errors and defects are reduced to the point of nearly being negligible.

Specificity: The proportion of patients without the target disorder who have a negative test result.

Stakeholder: An individual or entity that stands to lose or gain as a result of the research.

Standard deviation (SD): For a collection of observations, the SD represents the "average" deviation from the mean. It is the square root of the variance.

Standard error (SE): In multiple regression, the SE represents "average" deviation between actual and predicted observations. Graphically, it represents the spread or variability around the prediction line. Standard errors are also found for statistics, such as SE of the mean and SE for a proportion. In this context, the distribution of the sample means is normally shaped (bell shaped), regardless of the population from which the sample was obtained. The SE of the mean is the SD of the sample mean.

Standard error of the mean (SEM): This is the standard deviation (SD) divided by the square root of the sample size. It helps to quantify the precision of the mean by giving an indication of how far the sample mean is likely to be from the true population mean. The SEM is always smaller than the SD; in fact, with large samples, it is much smaller than the SD.

Systematic review: A high-quality summary of the literature that is based on explicit methods designed to accomplish a rigorous, comprehensive search and critical assessment of the included, individual studies. When appropriate statistical analysis is used on the pooled data, a quantitative systematic review, or meta-analysis, results.

t **distribution:** A theoretical relative frequency distribution in which the standard error of the mean is estimated from sample values; similar to a normal distribution but used when population variances are unknown.

t **test:** An *independent groups t test* is designed to compare means between 2 groups in which there are different subjects in each group. Ideally, the subjects are randomly selected from a larger population of subjects and assigned to 1 of 2 treatments. A *paired t test* is used when the subjects for the 2 groups are the same or matched, as in a pretest-posttest intervention.

Triple-blind study: The meaning of this term may vary but commonly indicates that the subject, researcher, and person administering the treatment are shielded from what is being given. Alternatively, it may mean that the patient, researcher, and data analyst are similarly shielded.

Two-tailed test: A statistical test in which the critical region for rejecting the null hypothesis falls in both directions of the probability distribution.

Type I error: Also called an "alpha (α) error." It occurs when the null hypothesis is falsely rejected; that is, researchers erroneously conclude that a difference exists between or among the treatment groups when, in fact, there is no difference.

Type II error: Also called a "beta (β) error." This type of error occurs when the null hypothesis is falsely accepted, that is, researchers erroneously conclude that no difference exists between or among the treatment groups when, in fact, there is a difference.

Validity: Refers to whether an instrument or a study truly measures what it was intended to measure or how truthful the research results are.

Variable: A value or quality than can vary between subjects or over time, or both.

Variance (S^2): Represents "average" squared deviations from the mean for a set of observations. Variances may be determined for linear combinations of observations as well.

Z distribution: A standard normal distribution; here it is the theoretical distribution of population scores in which the mean always equals 0 and the standard deviation equals 1.

Appendix. Electronic Databases for Searching the Literature

ACP Journal Club: A secondary journal of abstracts of articles containing strong evidence from the primary literature; from the American College of Physicians

CINAHL (Cumulative Index to Nursing & Allied Health Literature): Citations to systematic reviews

Cochrane Database of Systematic Reviews (full text), via Ovid: A collection of structured systematic reviews and protocols (which are systematic reviews in process)

Cochrane Database of Systematic Reviews (browse only, no full text): To browse Cochrane Systematic Reviews by topic and Cochrane Review Group

DARE (Database of Abstracts of Reviews of Effects): Abstracts of non-Cochrane systematic reviews

DynaMed: Evidence-based clinical review summaries

Embase: Access to current, comprehensive biomedical and drug information

Evidence-Based Medicine: Excellent secondary journal of high-quality research

Evidence-Based Perioperative Medicine: A superb international collaborative of institutions whose goal is to improve the outcome of patients having surgery

Medscape Reference (formerly eMedicine Clinical Knowledge Base): Background narratives, often with emphasis on best-evidence outcomes, covering topics across the medical and surgical spectrum

National Guideline Clearinghouse: Collection of guidelines from the Agency for Healthcare Research and Quality and professional medical societies

National Quality Measures Clearinghouse: Sponsored by Agency for Healthcare Research and Quality; a good source for structured, standardized abstracts and for information about measures and their development

Natural Standard: Graded evidence on complementary therapies

Ovid MEDLINE: Citations to systematic reviews

PubMed Clinical Queries: PubMed/MEDLINE search feature that filters results to display only articles backed by good evidence

TRIP Database: An evidence-based medicine search engine that searches across multiple evidence-based information sites; not all findings are full text, but includes many unique resources such as Bandolier and guidelines not found through the National Guideline Clearinghouse

UpToDate: Background narratives, often with emphasis on best evidence, with a special focus on internal medicine, family medicine, pediatrics, and obstetrics and gynecology

US Preventive Services Task Force: Database of evidence-based recommendations in areas of prevention and screening

Index to Figures

Index to Tables

Index to Appendices

About the Author

Chuck Biddle, CRNA, PhD, is a tenured full professor and staff anesthetist at Virginia Commonwealth University (VCU) in Richmond, Virginia. His earned doctorate is in the outcomes sciences of epidemiology. A nurse anesthetist for nearly 30 years, his research has always been grounded in the broad domain of patient safety and marshaling evidence-based decisions to the patient. He has been a university educator at several institutions during his career, including Old Dominion University, the University of Kansas, Dartmouth College, and, since 2000, VCU. Dr. Biddle serves as a reviewer for several peer-reviewed journals, has served as a reviewer for the anesthesia domain of The Cochrane Library, and has been Editor in Chief of the *AANA Journal* for 26 years. Dr. Biddle's peer-reviewed publication record has shown a consistent productivity throughout the course of his career, and he is fully committed to educating and mentoring those new to the field, as well as those who are experienced yet seek new pathways of enlightenment.